7507573792

Narrative therapy with couples ... and a whole lot more!

a collection of papers, essays and exercises

by

Jill Freedman & Gene Combs

AF756439

Dulwich Centre Publications
ADELAIDE, SOUTH AUSTRALIA

616
.89165
FRE

UNIVERSITY OF LEICESTER
UT VITAM HABEANT
LIBRARY

7507573792

ISBN 0 9577929 5 6

Copyright © 2002 by
Dulwich Centre Publications
Hutt St PO Box 7192
Adelaide 5000, South Australia
phone (61-8) 8223 3966, fax (61-8) 8232 4441
email: dcp@senet.com.au
website: www.dulwichcentre.com.au

Printed and manufactured by
Graphic Print Group, Richmond, South Australia.

The views expressed in this publication are not necessarily those of the Publisher. No part of this publication may be reproduced or transmitted by any process without the prior written permission of the Publisher.

Contents

Introduction

It is with great pleasure that we offer you this selection of papers and exercises. Many of these papers were written for large, multi-authored books. We have lamented that some of them might rarely be read by people who are immersed in narrative work - especially those papers written for books in which each chapter reflects a different model of therapy. We are grateful that these works are getting a second audience here. We are also pleased that this collection includes four exercises that we have developed - two in the section on exercises and one in the paper 'Gender Stories' and one in the paper 'Lists'. We think exercises can give people direct experience with the practices and implications of the narrative worldview. They are important tools for learning, but they are rarely published. We are glad that through this book more people will be able to use these exercises.

It is quite an experience to read back over these papers all at once. They reflect a "history of the present" for us. They take us back to experiences in particular rooms, to specific conversations where new ideas and practices were born; they help us re-member turning points in our stories of therapy and life.

Although we would write some things differently now than we did in our earlier papers, we are pleasantly surprised to discover what we were on to way back then! One difference we notice is that where we once thought in terms of social constructionism, we are now finding that post-structuralism offers ideas and images that let us more clearly articulate the politics of this work. We do not regret our study of social constructionism. In engaging with that school of thought we were able to deconstruct for ourselves many structuralist notions about identity. This has contributed significantly to all of our work.

Acknowledgements

In revisiting these papers, we also revisit those people who contributed most significantly to them. Writing the "Minimizing Hierarchy" paper with Michele Cohen, David Larimer, Pat DeLaurenti, Bill DeLaurenti, and Dina Shulman was a wonderful experience we will always treasure. We are grateful to all the authors of that paper. Writing the children's article with Jenny Simons was a more formal way to revisit the talks about the ins and outs of working with young people that we have had the good fortune of sharing with her over the years. We are better therapists for participating in this collaboration.

We probably wouldn't have written any of these papers if people hadn't continually supported our teaching. This includes the various organizations, agencies, and clinics who have sponsored us over the years and all the people who have come to workshops and classes when they were offered. The ideas that appear here in print were shaped by our interactions with people in those settings. All of these papers rely on the experience of working with specific people at poignant moments in their lives. We very much appreciate the people who open their lives to us and trust us with their stories.

Because of the lighthearted way both David Denborough and Cheryl White approach serious matters, the making of this book has been a delightful experience – as always, it has been a joy to work with them. We'd also like to acknowledge Jane Hales for her layout skills and Chris McLean, Leonie Thomas and Ian Thomas for their proofreading. Finally, we'd like to thank Michael White and David Epston, whose ideas have changed our lives.

1. Jill and Gene can be contacted at the Evanston Family Therapy Center, 636 Church Street, #901, Evanston, Illinois 60201, USA, phone: (1-847) 866 7879, fax: (1-847) 328 1212.

PART ONE

Working with couples

1

Placing couple work in context [1]

Working with couples is something we thoroughly enjoy. It is a significant aspect of our professional life. People in heterosexual relationships regularly request to see us together so that therapists of both genders are represented in the room, while perhaps a third of my (JF) therapy is with lesbian couples. As we are in an intimate relationship ourselves, having lived together and been married for a long time, this informs our work with couples in many ways. Our own relationship adds to our commitment to working with people in intimate partnerships. At the same time, it means we must try not to make assumptions about other people's lives based on our own experiences.

In this short paper, we have tried to outline some of the powerful discourses about couples and intimate relationships in the culture in which we live, and some of the hazards and possibilities these discourses produce. To begin though, we'd like to articulate some of the reasons why we believe so-called 'couple' work is a significant and important area of practice.

Why work with 'couples' is significant to us

Over the years, we have witnessed various inadvertent affects of individual therapy and this has led us to a strong commitment to involving significant others in counseling contexts wherever possible. For instance, I (JF) can remember a woman, whom I shall refer to here as Veronique, who had been in individual therapy for many years to address the effects of sexual abuse that she had experienced in childhood. Veronique was in a long-term relationship with Juan, and they were parenting two young children. After some years of individual therapy, their relationship broke down. I recall both Veronique and Juan speaking of their regrets, saying that if Juan had been involved in some way in the therapy process - as a witness to the steps Veronique was taking, or as an active support person in some other way - then their relationship may well have remained strong. It was the construction of therapy as an individually oriented process that in some ways contributed to separating Veronique and Juan. They both expressed sadness about this, as did their children.

While we both still offer individual therapy, we now believe that linking such therapy to the broader relationships in a person's life is highly significant. We now always enquire as to the effects of therapy on a person's other relationships and ask about including particularly significant people in the therapy process in some way. This might mean inviting these significant others into the therapy room as witnesses, or involving them through documents or rituals either during the therapy process or at its completion. In the culture in which we live, when we are working with adults, this often means working with partners in some way, although significant others can also include friends, siblings, work mates, children, parents, grandparents and other significant people from a particular community.

The catalyst for many men to show up for therapy with me (GC) is the encouragement from their female partners to seek help. In these instances, it feels important to me to involve the woman partner in some way, at least initially. When the impetus for therapy has come from someone else, I always want to at least meet this other person so I can hear from them directly why they believe therapy is a relevant step, rather than following my own assumptions about this. Sometimes this leads to ongoing work with both members of the 'couple', other times it simply creates a solid platform from which to begin working with the particular man.

Of course, much of our work with intimate partners/couples occurs when we are approached because of certain difficulties that are occurring within the relationship itself. In the culture in which we live, couple relationships are a key place where people find and create intimacy, love, trust and commitment. These relationships are one of the principal realms of meaning making and identity. This means that many people spend a good deal of time in couple relationships and addressing any difficulties within these relationships is a high priority.

Cultural discourses about 'couples' and 'coupling'

While we wish to honour the significance that intimate couple relationships play in so many people's lives, it seems important to acknowledge that there is much about the culture in which we live that privileges 'couple' relationships over other forms of relating. There are powerful discourses that influence this premium that is placed on 'couples' and 'coupling.' These discourses shape people's understandings about what intimate relationships should look like. They set specifications for couple relationships in terms of appropriate intimacy, length of relationship, ways of communicating, degree of romance, sexual arrangements and many other things. There are also broader cultural discourses which promote the idea that couple relationships ought to be heterosexual and between people of similar ages, social status, and race. In the US at this time these discourses are inextricably linked to a strong conservative 'family values' campaign that promotes a particular vision of the heterosexual Christian nuclear family. The word 'couple' in this context can disqualify or disempower sole-parent families, as well as other kinds of relationships. All of these discourses powerfully influence people's experiences of their relationships. It seems important to acknowledge that this is the broader social and political context of our work with 'couples'.

There are all sorts of subtle and not so subtle ways in which we as therapists can collude with dominant discourses around couples and relationships. For instance, we can recall a recent consultation with a man, Steve, who is in midlife and who, for a range of reasons, has reached a decision not to be involved in an intimate or 'couple' relationship. This was an important and empowering decision for Steve - one which he clearly stated that he felt very good about. However, when a team of therapists then offered reflections on this interview one member of the team spoke of how sad she felt about Steve's decision. This is an example of how we as therapists are powerfully influenced by dominant understandings of what a 'good' or 'happy' life should look like. There is a strong cultural discourse that encourages us to believe that people are somehow 'incomplete' if they are not in a conventional couple relationship. It seems to us that we need to take great care in this work not to privilege couple relationships over other relationships and ways of living.

For that matter, framing this work as 'couples therapy' can be somewhat problematic in itself. The notion of couple therapy can invite us as therapists to consider that problems reside somehow within 'the couple' whereas they may instead be due to broader socio-cultural factors, or even in some instances to the dominant definitions of 'coupledom' which can place unsustainable limits on relationships.

For instance, I (JF) am reminded of Vanessa, whose partner, Phil, has been ill for more than 10 years. Vanessa has declared to me on many occasions her love for Phil and her wish to stay by his side. However, Vanessa is also lamenting that it has not been possible to have a sexual relationship with Phil for a decade. Vanessa wants to remain married and yet also longs for a sexual relationship and/or sexual experiences. Her belief, and it is certainly not hers alone, is that it is not possible for her to have a sexual relationship outside of her marriage and still to honour her marriage. It is this combination of her sexual longing and her beliefs about what is honourable in marriage that is creating the considerable distress that Vanessa is experiencing. The problem is not between her and Phil; yet Vanessa is having fantasies of leaving their marriage. She has said to me that leaving Phil entirely would in some ways be more possible than ever being able to have a conversation about, or entertain possibilities of, having some sort of sexual relationship while still in their marriage.

The dominant construction of 'couple therapy' also encourages the idea that only the two people who are in an intimate relationship should be seen in the therapy room. This invites us to cast our focus solely upon the couple and their relationship when there may be far more creative and generative places to look and areas in which to take action.

Some time ago, we were members of a reflecting team for a heterosexual couple who were talking about how they lived in a set of apartments in which different family members and different couples would all come together to eat their evening meals. The woman of this particular couple was speaking to us about how she felt that there must be something wrong with their couple relationship because they had a great time whenever they were eating in this more collective manner, and yet when they ate dinner just with the two of them they didn't have such an enjoyable time. To this woman this was indicative that there must be something wrong with their relationship. Upon further exploration however, we all came to realise that it was instead a vivid example of some of the effects of normalising judgments in relation to 'couple' life. In this instance, as in the story told above, the problem was not within the relationship but in the dominant construction of what intimate relationships should be.

We are all born into, and live within, cultural stories that are not always visible to us. When we meet with people who believe there is something problematic about the ways in which they are relating to each other, we are very interested in unpacking the context for the problems they are experiencing. We want to create the possibility for people to articulate what is it that they might be measuring their relationship against, and what types of cultural ideas their notions of relationship are situated within. In turn, we wish to make it possible for people to begin to clearly articulate the values which they wish to inform their relationships and their reasons for choosing those values. We want to create a context where people can unpack their assumptions about relationships and richly describe what is important to them and why. We hope to enable people to more consciously shape their relationships, rather than to collude in some way with normative specifications.

One of the reasons that I (JF) really appreciate working with people in gay and lesbian relationships is that, by definition, these relationships do not fit the dominant model. People living lesbian and gay lives are often more able to examine some of this culture's taken-for-granted notions of relationship and make their own decisions about how they wish to relate to those they care about. People in lesbian and gay relationships are often more conscious about the active process of making and re-forming family. Their perspectives on these issues continue to influence our work with heterosexual couples as well as our own lives.

While strongly committed to not reproducing normative ideas in our work, we are part of the dominant culture, and subject to the discourses about 'coupledom' that we outlined above. For instance, I (GC) enter any therapy discussion as a man who is in a loving and satisfying heterosexual couple relationship. While I have chosen this lifestyle, and am very pleased with it, I am also conscious that broader cultural discourses have shaped my choices. Our relationship is based on an agreement of monogamy, and we are the parents of a child. In any therapy session I have to work hard to ensure I am not assuming that what works for me is going to make anyone else happy. As our lifestyle choices largely fit with the dominant discourses of the culture, this makes questioning our assumptions all the more relevant.

This questioning, of course, is one of the key characteristics of narrative work. There are a range of questions that we find helpful to consistently ask ourselves:

- What am I tending to assume here?
- How might my gender be influencing what I am attending to and what I am not attending to?
- How might my experience as someone in a heterosexual monogamous relationship be influencing what I'm hearing and what I'm saying?
- Am I in any way imposing my beliefs about what intimate relationships should look like?
- How can I clarify the preferences, beliefs and values that the people consulting me hold about their relationship?
- How can I provide the opportunity to those consulting me to unpack their own assumptions about their relationships?

We couldn't possibly list all the assumptions which therapists and those consulting therapists hold about relationships and couples, but one of the major areas in which assumptions need to be unpacked is around practices of gender. While this is often relevant to gay and lesbian couples, it is almost always a key aspect of work with heterosexual couples, as patriarchal assumptions are so powerfully taken for granted in our culture. When patriarchal assumptions are taken for granted, they can bring forth power inequities and make violence seem justified. We do not directly address working with violence and abuse in this section, but it is an important aspect of this work. For an example of how we work with violence in couple relationships, see 'Relationships and Ethics' in the Essays section of this book.

The joys of this work

Having outlined some of the complexities of this work, we would like to briefly describe what we particularly appreciate about working with couples. The ways in which narrative work engages one person in a conversation while the other listens before reflecting, can create a beautiful rhythm when working with couples. It is our job to create a context for each partner to witness the stories of the other in new and different ways. In turn, this creates possibilities for change and healing and we thoroughly enjoy this process. When couples work is going well, after problems have been externalised and their broader social context deconstructed, we get to hear stories of how each partner has helped the other to articulate and realise their dreams, their hopes, and their successes in becoming more the person they want to be in the partnership. We get to hear about shared ideals and directions in life and witness these becoming more richly articulated and performed. It can be quite joyous to participate in these conversations - even if those in the couple decide that their relationship needs to change significantly.

There are further reasons why we greatly appreciate working with couples; perhaps these are best illustrated with one final story. Rosie, is an older woman who has multiple sclerosis. She can't walk and has many physical limitations. Milton, Rosie's long term partner, has recently died. Actually, he was more than a partner; Milton was also Rosie's primary caregiver. He fulfilled this role willingly and with great love. Since Milton's death there has been a process in which Rosie is only now realising that she requires help. She is only now recognising her individual limitations. While everybody else knew that there were things Rosie needed help with, as long as she and Milton were together, she didn't experience her own limits. In fact, in the context of their relationship, she did not have those limitations. While Milton and Rosie were together, those limitations simply did not exist.

We have both found this somewhat miraculous. For me (JF) it is has been particularly moving because Rosie is my mother and Milton was my father. It is only now that my mother is saying, 'I realise that I can't be alone at night'. This means that for years and years she hasn't known this.

In some cultures, people's identities are formed largely and continually in community, and people's individual selves are not so profoundly separated from extended family and communal life. But in the individualistic culture in which we live, intimate couple relationships are one of the few places in which we move beyond our bounded individualities. They are one of the few places where the dissolution of individual selves takes place. To us, this means that these relationships are both precious and pressured. And it makes providing a place for people to talk about these relationships all the more important.

Note

1. This article was created from an interview conducted by David Denborough at our home in Evanston in February 2002.

2

Narrative couple therapy

This chapter was originally published in Gurman & Jacobson's (2002) Clinical Handbook of Couple Therapy. *We were specifically requested by the editors to organise this paper under certain categories. While we would not have chosen these categories, we believe this paper lays out some of the key principles of narrative practice with couples.*

We were also asked as part of the initial publishing request to provide a lengthy example of work with one couple. In this paper, and in the other three papers in this section of the book, the examples of work described are with heterosexual couples. This is partly because of the context of the initial requests, and also due to some reluctance on our part as heterosexual therapists to write about the lives and relationships of lesbian and gay couples.

With these provisos in mind, we believe this following paper offers a thorough reflection on our work with couples and gives a glimmer of the complexities involved.

Background

'Narrative therapy', as we (Freedman & Combs 1996) use the term, refers to a growing body of practices and ideas (Freeman, Epston & Lobovits 1997; Monk, Winslade, Crocket & Epston 1997; Morgan 2000; Zimmerman & Dickerson 1996) that stem from the work of Michael White and David Epston. White's early published work (e.g. 1986) was based on ideas that stem from the work of Gregory Bateson (1972). David Epston (1989, 1998), who had encountered the narrative metaphor in studying anthropology, and Cheryl White, 'who had enthusiasm for this analogy from her readings in feminism'(White & Epston 1990, p.xvi) encouraged White to use the 'story analogy' – the notion that meaning is constituted through the stories we tell and hear concerning our lives. In collaboration with Epston, White (White & Epston 1990, 1992) found that the story analogy offered a useful direction for their work.

Therapists who began to use the narrative metaphor in White's and Epston's sense experienced quite a large shift in their worldview. Instead of trying to solve problems, they became interested in collaborating with people to change their lives through enriching the narratives they and others tell concerning their lives. They began to work to bring forth and develop 'thick descriptions' (Geertz 1978; Ryle 1990, 1971) or rich, meaningful, multistranded stories of those aspects of people's life narratives that lie outside the influence of problems. It seems that through these alternative stories, people can live out new identities, new possibilities for relationship, and new futures.

This work is more complex than a brief description of the narrative metaphor might suggest. One factor adding to the complexity is that some stories have more staying power than others. In any culture at any given time, certain stories are much more a part of the fabric of day-to-day reality than are others. We are all born into cultural stories, and they shape our perceptions of what is possible. For couples, stories about gender roles and heterosexual dominance, for example, may shape perceptions of what is possible. However, people do not usually think of the stories they are born into as stories. They think of them as 'reality'. Cultural stories have the power to shape our experience of reality.

An important influence on how narrative therapists work with the stories that circulate in people's cultures has been 'poststructuralism', especially as it is expressed in the late work of Michel Foucault (1980, 1985). Foucault was a

French intellectual who studied, among other things, the various ways that people in Western society have been categorized as 'other'. He examined madness (1965), illness (1975), criminality (1977), and sexuality (1985) as concepts around which certain people have been labeled 'insane', 'sick', 'criminal', or 'perverted', and described various ways such people have been separated, oppressed, or enrolled in self-policing on the basis of that labeling.

To Foucault, people have power in a society in direct proportion to their ability to participate in the various discourses that shape that society. Although *The American Heritage Dictionary, Third Edition* gives simply 'verbal expression in speech or writing' as its first definition of 'discourse', scholars like Foucault use the word to refer to the ongoing political/historical/institutional conversations within a society that constitute our notions of what is true and what is possible. Foucault showed how the people whose voices dominated the discussion about what constituted madness, for example, could separate the people *they* saw as mad from 'polite society', sequestering them in madhouses where their voices were cut off from the avenues of power.

Foucault argued that there is an inseparable linkage between knowledge and power. Because the discourses of a society determine what knowledge is held to be true, right, or proper in that society, those who control the discourse control knowledge. At the same time, the dominant knowledge of a given milieu determines who will be able to occupy its powerful positions. We see the discourses of power that Foucault studied as historical, cultural metanarratives – stories that have shaped (and been shaped by) the distribution of power in society.

Society is not necessarily benign, fair, or just. As feminist critics (e.g. Avis 1985; Carter, Papp, Silverstein & Walters 1984; Goldner 1985a, 1985b; Hare-Mustin 1978; Laird 1989; Taggart 1985) of family therapy have reminded us, our cultural institutions constrain us, leading us to see certain possibilities as desirable and blinding us to other possibilities. Laird (1989, p.430) writes that 'sociocultural narratives ... construct the contextual realms of possibility from which individuals and families can select the ingredients and forms for their own narratives'. Some people have readier access to a wider range of sociocultural narratives than others, and some narratives dominate while others are marginalized. Laird (1989, p.431) reminds of this when she writes of '... the politics of storymaking or mythmaking. Clearly there are both obvious and subtle differences in the power individuals and particular interest groups possess to ensure that particular narratives will prevail in family, group, and national life. Not all stories are equal.'

Socially constructed narratives have real effects. For example, the myth that 'welfare mothers' are engaged in a mini-industry in which they get richer and richer as they make more and more babies has had real effects on already undeserved women and children. It has provided a rationalization that has allowed those in power to cut funds even further. The story about how women can never be too thin which gets retold every time one turns on the TV or stands in a supermarket checkout line surrounded by magazine covers displaying anorexia nervosa as beauty[1], has contributed to a real epidemic of self-starvation. The widely circulated stories in which inner-city males are only interested in drugs, sex, and killing each other support the perverse glorification of certain kinds of misogyny and violence. At the same time, they have served as a rationale for giving up on social policies that might offer inner-city males a real chance at a different way of making it in the world.

Foucault was especially interested in how the 'truth claims' carried in the 'grand abstractions' of reductionist science constitutes a discourse that dehumanizes and objectifies many people. He was interested in finding and circulating marginalized discourses – stories that exist, but are not widely circulated or powerfully endorsed – that might undermine the excessive power of the reductionistic scientific discourse. Foucault (1980) wrote of the 'amazing efficacy of discontinuous, particular, and local criticism' (p.80) in bringing about a 'return of knowledge' or 'an insurrection of subjugated knowledges' (p.84).

Following Foucault, we believe that even in the most marginalized and disempowered of lives, there is always lived experience that lies outside the dominant stories. White, Epston, and other narrative therapists have developed ways of thinking and working that bring forth the 'discontinuous, particular, and local' stories of couples and other social groups, so that people can inhabit and lay claim to the many possibilities for their lives that lie beyond the pale of dominant narratives.

When we use the narrative metaphor and the lens of poststructuralism to orient our work as therapists, we are intensely curious about each new couple we meet. We cherish each couple's stories. We work with the partners in couples in ways that invite them to celebrate their differences and to develop and live out narratives that they prefer around the particularities of their lives. This valuing of the meaning people make of their own experience over the meaning experts make of that experience has been referred to as the 'interpretive turn' (Bruner 1986). It leads us to de-center our meanings and to experience ourselves as interested people – perhaps with an anthropological or biographical or field researcher's bent – who are skilled at asking questions to bring forth the knowledge and experience carried in the stories of the couples we work with. We work to help people notice the influence of restrictive cultural stories in their lives, and to expand and enrich their own life narratives. We strive to find ways to spread the news of triumphs – to circulate success stories in order to keep them alive and growing. We believe that these success stories in turn contribute to keeping our culture growing and flowing in satisfying ways.

The healthy/well-functioning vs pathological/dysfunctional couple/marriage

'Healthy', 'well-functioning', 'pathological', and 'dysfunctional' are not descriptions we generally use. If we are to think in this language, whether couples are 'well-functioning' or not has to do with whether the stories they are living and in which they construct their identities are ones that they prefer. We think of relationships as being multi-storied. That is, every relationship can be expressed and experienced through a great variety of narratives; many 'true' stories can be told about any experience. Therefore, we do not look for health or pathology or quality of functioning in couples. Instead, we look at the stories that are currently shaping a relationship, and seek to facilitate a collaborative re-authoring process in which more suitable stories can be expressed and experienced.

Similarly, we do not consider the partners in a couple to have essential, core identities with fixed, predictable characteristics. Therefore, we do not look for 'health' or 'pathology' within the members of a couple. Keeping in mind the interpretive turn, we are interested in people's evaluations of what is problematic and preferred, and of how the problems they name affect their lives and relationships. That we are interested in people making their own evaluations does not mean that we think anything goes. We are full participants in the process of therapy, and we inevitably bring our own opinions and hard-won lived experience (and biases) along with us. For example, we are opposed to (among other things) abuse, coercion, and cruelty. When one of these problems appears to have invaded a relationship, we consider it our responsibility to ask questions that invite each partner to consider the effects of the problem on his/her life, the other partner's life, and their relationship, and to consider the stand he/she wants to take in relation to it.

We seek to create a conversational space in which people can take responsibility for addressing and ameliorating the effects of, for instance, abuse. To us, this means that we must avoid lecturing or imposing rigid rules from a position of moral superiority. Instead, we want to invite people to bring their 'best selves' into a consideration of the ways abuse diminishes their relationship, and an exploration of how they might choose ways of living that keep the abuse out of their relationship.

As narrative therapists, one of our principal intentions is to subvert the dominant practice in our society of measuring ourselves, our relationships, and others by standardized norms. For us, two-dimensional normative scales ('healthy–sick', 'gifted–impaired', etc.) invite therapists and the couples who consult with them into thin descriptions – pallid, reductionist accounts – of their multi-storied lives. These two-dimensional scales pervade contemporary Western culture, and each of them co-exists with a prescriptive story about the right or healthy or successful way to live or to have a relationship. And none of us can measure up to the demands of all these norms; we are too fat or too thin, too driven or too passive, too caring or not caring enough. Our relationships are too rigid or too enmeshed, too focused on sex or not sexy enough, too hot or too cold. Even when we do measure up, it is within the dictates of a thin, two-dimensional story.

Rather than looking for pathology or flawed functioning within couples, we seek to examine problematic cultural stories in collaborative and multi-dimensional ways. We engage in conversations to expose problematic discourses and give couples the opportunity to describe and evaluate the effects of those discourses on their relationship. For example, let us discuss a conversation we had with Ted and Carol. Carol complained that Ted always walked ahead of her, and at malls always led them into the stores he wanted to shop in, not the ones she would prefer. When Carol noticed this pattern, she wondered whether it meant that she was a slow person or that Ted did not care about her and her preferences. Ted thought that all it meant was that he was a fast walker. As we asked questions to explore the cultural stories that shaped their way of walking, it seemed to all of us that gender socialization had supported Ted in unthinkingly setting the pace and Carol in unthinkingly following along, even though it made her feel like a 'little girl' or a 'puppy dog'. Our conversation allowed Carol and Ted to separate themselves from the problem, notice the effects it had on their lives, and consider what they would prefer for their relationship.

We have worked with couples in which corporate values have played the largest role in creating problems, keeping one member of the couple unavailable and inattentive to what was most important both to him or herself and to the relationship. In the couple we describe later in this chapter, differences in social class contributed to problematic power relations and bred fear and doubt in the relationship. In each instance, the stories about what discourses were negatively influencing their relationship, and about their preferred directions in life, emerged in collaborative conversation with a couple. Our desires in each instance were for the couple to have the last word as to what was preferred, and for the choices to be made within a multi-dimensional domain, not against a two-dimensional yardstick.

The assessment of couple functioning and dysfunction

We think about information as being *generated* rather than 'gathered' in therapeutic conversations. In a rather literal way, we believe that we are making ourselves and each other up as we go along. This is a poststructuralist idea. We do not assume that a couple has a particular interactional or relational structure that we can assess. We do not think of people or relationships as having stable, quantifiable identities or 'typical' characteristics, so we do not try to discover or gather information about such characteristics. Instead, we think of people's lives as being multistoried, and we believe that each new telling generates new possibilities for interpretation and action.

Although we avoid the position of making professional, 'expert' assessments, we acknowledge that the role of therapist/interviewer is a powerful one. Each question we ask directs attention to a particular domain and away from many others. We want people to interpret and assess their own experience, but our questions inevitably shape the inquiry. For this reason, we 'situate' our questions. That is, we describe where they come from and our intentions in asking them so that people can evaluate our bias and decide how to relate to it. We believe that people are in a better position to interpret, make meaning of, and assess their own experience than outsiders are, even outsiders trained to help.

Since we do not subscribe to normative ideas of what constitutes a healthy couple relationship, we would be at a loss about what criteria to use in assessing couples. Instead of assessment, we are interested in hearing detailed, context-specific narratives. As we ask questions to bring forth their stories, we encourage those with whom we work to evaluate problems and their relationship to problems, as well as evaluating the therapy itself.

We ask questions that invite the partners in a couple to do the following:

- assess their current situation,
- name the problems involved,
- evaluate their relationship to those problems,
- take a stand in regard to them,
- tell more satisfying stories of their relationship,
- assess the usefulness of the alternative stories.

We want to know whether the alternative stories speak to people of a more satisfying identity as a couple. In telling the new stories and reflecting on them, people collaborate with us in an ongoing assessment of their new expressions of themselves and their relationship.

Here are some questions we might ask in inviting people's assessments of their situation and of their therapy experience:

- 'What name would you give the problem?'
- 'What is it like to have the experience of the problem?'
- 'What effect does the problem have on your life?'
- 'What effect does the problem have on your relationship with each other?'
- 'What has it talked you into about your partner? What impact has that had?'

- 'What effect does the problem have on other relationships?'
- 'How does the problem alter your relationship with yourself?'
- 'Is this what you want for your relationship? Why or why not?'
- 'Is this what you want for yourself? Why or why not?'
- 'Are we talking about what you want to be talking about?'
- 'Is this conversation useful?'
- 'How is it useful?'

In telling and living out the many strands of alternative stories, the partners in a couple evaluate many aspects of their lives: their private thoughts, feelings, hopes, and fears; their dyadic interactions; the contributions of each partner's culture of origin to the couple and to the individual partners; their interrelationship with local institutions and traditions; and more.

Although we bend over backward to avoid 'expert', categorical, reductionist assessment, it would be misleading to imply that we make no assessments of any kind. One kind of assessment that we make has to do with which parts of a couple's story might be shaped by discourses that are invisible to the partners. We ask questions that invite them to unmask the operations of such discourses, and that offer an opportunity to decide where they stand and how they would like their relationship to be in the face of such discourses.

We are particularly interested in bringing forth partners' evaluations of power relations. This often involves asking questions that invite them to consider the effects of discourses of gender, ethnicity, heterosexual dominance, class, corporate culture, patriarchy, age, or other sociocultural factors on their relationship. We might initiate such a conversation with questions similar to those that follow. We try to have thoughtful interactive conversations, with each question being responsive to the last answer. It is difficult to capture that flavor in a series of hypothetical questions. We would not ask these questions in the beginning of a conversation. They would follow a detailed telling of a set of experiences.

- *Martha, you have just said that fear of humiliation keeps you from wanting to go to social events with Brian. You described his failure to introduce you to people he knows and his talking over you when you try to join in. Is that right?*
- *Brian, what is it like to hear your actions being described that way? Does it fit with how you like to think of yourself?*
- *What or who do you think might have introduced you to this way of acting?*
- *Your father and uncles undoubtedly did not make up this way of being. Where do you think they might have learned it?*
- *Martha, I've noticed that all of these examples are of men. Do you think that this is a coincidence?*
- *Do you think it is a way of acting only to women or to children as well?*
- *What should we call this way of acting?*
- *Brian, what do you think it might be like to be a woman or child experiencing discounting?*
- *Is this what you would want women and children to experience from you? Why not? What would you rather have them know about you?*
- *You have already said, Martha, that this discounting keeps you from wanting to socialize with John. Are there other ways it affects your relationship?*
- *Is this what you want for your relationship? What would you prefer?*
- *We've been talking about a strand of our culture in which women and children are invisible or are considered to be property. It is clear, John, that that does not fit with your thinking, although you have gotten pulled into some ways of acting that go with it. Martha, do you think you've been pulled into some of the actions that go with these ideas as well?*
- *What would you name them?*
- *What's that been like for you?*
- *What has it been like for the relationship, do you think? How would you prefer your relationship to be?*

Because we think that 'self', 'identity', 'personhood', and the like are experiences that emerge and are always changing *in relationship*, we do not know exactly who will be answering when we ask a person to draw a distinction or to evaluate the effect of an action. To make this transparent, we might ask, 'Is that the problem speaking?' or 'Whose values are guiding you in saying that – gay culture's or straight culture's?'

In exposing discourses that support problems, individuals and couples can separate themselves from the ways of being that are supported by those discourses, and can identify and recognize preferred perceptions, attitudes, and actions. Although we do not think of strengths or resources as fixed commodities, and we do not administer questionnaires to inventory them, we are very interested to hear the stories of relationships and events that help people to have a sense of choice, agency, purpose, and accomplishment in their life as a couple.

Goal-setting

Our general goal in therapy is to collaborate with people in living out moment-by-moment, choice-by-choice life stories that they prefer, that are more just, and that make their worlds more satisfying. We are more interested in opening up possibilities than we are in closing them down. This makes us wary of 'goal-setting' as it is usually defined and practiced. We think that goals, unless they are very tentatively set and rigorously updated, can set single, specific trajectories for people's lives. This can all too easily close down possibilities. The narrative metaphor biases us toward thinking about possibilities that unfold in living out a story, rather than about goals, which are usually set in advance and pursued more-or-less single-mindedly. Instead of goals, we tend to speak of 'projects' or 'directions in life'.

The process of identifying projects is fluid, shifting as new distinctions are made and as alternative stories unfold. Problems can be thought of as plots and projects as counterplots. Partners in a couple may name joint projects for the relationship, individual projects, or both. For some couples, the collaborative negotiation of shared or complementary directions in life can be a very significant – sometimes even an inspirational – part of the therapy.

The structure of the therapy process

Although we take an active role in structuring the therapy, we ask couples to collaborate with us so that the process will fit their circumstances.

Telling and witnessing

A rhythmic alternation between telling and witnessing characterizes narrative work. We set up a structure early in our work with couples that we come back to over and over again. We ask one member of the couple to tell his or her story while the other listens from a witnessing position. Then we ask the witnesser to reflect on what he or she has heard. Next we switch positions, so that the partner who had been in the witnessing position can tell his or her story.

We initiate this process by making eye contact and speaking primarily with one person at a time, then asking the partner to comment. Sometimes we are more explicit, saying something like this: 'What I would like to do is speak with you, Rubin, for a time, with you, Ellen, listening. After a bit I'll turn to you, Ellen, and ask what thoughts you have been having while Rubin has been talking. Then we'll switch and you, Rubin, will be in the listening position while Ellen and I have a conversation. Would that be OK?'

We use the alternation of telling and witnessing in other ways as well. Sometimes a couple describes something and the therapist reflects. Although the two of us most often work separately, many people know us to be partners in marriage and in parenthood as well as in our work. Heterosexual couples in particular sometimes ask us to work with them as a co-therapy team. When we do this, one of us takes the role of interviewer and the other reflects. Sometimes we include an outsider witness group or reflecting team as part of the structure. In that case, the outsider witness group listens while we interview the couple. Then we have a formal break and the outsider witnesses reflect on what they've heard. In the last part of the interview, the couple responds to the reflections. At times, particularly as part of training or consultation, reflecting teams are composed of therapists. At other times, in response to our raising the possibility, couples agree to our inviting another couple (whose members have insider experience in dealing with a particular problem) to serve as an outsider witness group. Or couples may invite other people who are important in their lives to join in as an outsider witness group.

Length, frequency, and number of meetings

We negotiate the time of each next meeting as we go along, one session at a time. At the end of meetings with couples, we ask whether the conversation has been useful. If it has, we ask how. Then we ask whether they would like to meet again, and if so, when.

We ask couples to make these decisions each time, so that they are at least as active as we are in evaluating what schedule would be most useful. Sometimes, as when they are in the middle of intense conversations, couples want to return very soon. More often, because partners have been hearing each other in new ways and making new distinctions, they are interested in allowing some time to find out what difference these new experiences will make in their lives. We listen as they negotiate with each other about how long their explorations will take. Occasionally, because the partners are not sure how much time would be useful, a couple decides to telephone us for the next appointment.

We generally meet with couples for 60 minutes at a time, but have negotiated longer meeting times for future meetings when we all agreed that we wished there was more time to complete a conversation. How long therapy lasts is highly variable and determined by each couple. Some couples come to deal with a single problem, and therapy may consist of two or three meetings. Others become involved in developing very rich, detailed stories of the partners' lives together. Their therapy may continue for several years. Most are somewhere in-between.

Focusing on new directions in life

We wonder whether simply sitting down for a meeting in a therapy office invites people to re-immerse themselves in problematic stories. With this in mind, we structure therapy conversations so as to invite people to continue to explore, describe, and experience directions in life that were unfolding in our previous meetings – new distinctions, positions people have taken about their relationship to problems, and new stories that are developing. Sometimes we read our notes aloud and ask a question such as: 'Can you tell us about new developments that relate to what we were talking about last time?' Sometimes we begin by wondering whether there have been important thoughts or events that connect to our conversation of the time before.

Another way we structure therapy is through thinking about how to keep stories alive and growing between conversations. We use letters, documents, videotapes, and the like to document and circulate alternative stories. For example, after a therapy interview we may write a letter posing questions that invite the partners to develop an alternative story even farther than they had in the interview, or we may send a document noting the stands they have taken in regard to a problem. We think that the reading of such a document between therapy meetings and the conversations that may follow such a reading can contribute to keeping a story alive and growing.

Medication

Our experience is that ideas about medication are so pervasive that the people who come to us for therapy raise the issue before it ever occurs to us. Medications are rarely a focus of couple therapy. If something about one partner's medication or the condition for which it is being prescribed does seem to be problematic for a couple, we address that problem in the same manner that we address other problems – asking each partner to describe the problem and its effects, identifying 'unique outcomes' (those events that stand outside of and would not be predicted by the problem story) concerning the problem, and developing the stories of those unique outcomes.

The role of the therapist

Epston (1999, pp.141-142) writes:

> *I chose to orient myself around the co-research metaphor both because of its beguiling familiarity and because it radically departed from conventional clinical practice. It brought together the very respectable notion of research with the rather odd idea of the co-production of knowledge by sufferers and therapist ... This has led, and continually leads, to practices to discover a "knowing" in such a fashion that all parties to it could make good use of it. Such knowledges are fiercely and unashamedly pragmatic.*

We join Epston in thinking of our work as co-research.

In order to engage in co-research, the therapeutic relationship is extremely important. As co-researchers, we have more questions than answers about therapeutic relationships. The following are some questions we (Freedman & Combs, 2000) ask ourselves so that we can adjust our participation in relationships with couples as therapy goes along:

- Whose voice is being privileged in this relationship? What is the effect of that on the relationship and the work?
- Is anyone showing signs of being closed down, not able to fully enter into the work? If so, what power relations/discourses are contributing to the closing down?
- What are we doing to foster collaboration? Among whom? What is the effect of that collaboration?
- Is this relationship opening up or closing down the experience of agency?
- Does this relationship take into account other relevant people, communities, and cultures? Are we considering the effects of the ripples of this relationship?
- Am I asking whether and how the work is useful, and tailoring it in line with the response?

White (2000) describes a therapist's role in this work as de-centered, but influential. We participate not as representatives of professional knowledge, not as authorities on what constitutes a normal or healthy relationship, but as people with skills in facilitating a co-research project.

We ask questions to help expose gaps or contradictions in the problematic stories that bring couples to therapy and to open space for and thickly describe alternatives. We work to keep the conversation focused and relevant. We facilitate people's ongoing evaluation of the process by asking how the conversation is going for them and responding to their answers. At times, we reflect and offer alternative directions for our conversations.

We work to create a collaborative context. We situate our ideas in our own experience and make our intentions transparent. We encourage couples to ask questions about our questions and comments. When therapy goes well (and sometimes even when it does not), we all change. We acknowledge to couples how our work and lives are enriched through meeting with them.

Techniques of couple therapy

Listening

When we meet people for the first time, we want to understand the meaning of their stories for *them*. This means turning our backs on 'expert' filters: not listening for chief complaints; not 'gathering' the pertinent-to-us-as-experts bits of diagnostic information interspersed in their stories; not hearing their anecdotes as matrices within which resources are embedded; not listening for surface hints about what the core problem 'really' is; and not comparing the selves they portray in their stories to normative standards.

In the beginning, we ask about non-problematic aspects of the lives of each partner and of their relationship. We are interested in getting to know the members of a couple as people, and in making sure that the problem does not trick us into mistaking them for it. Unless people insist on moving quickly into talking about problems, we spend a while listening to stories about their preferences and pleasures. At some point in this process, people do usually begin to spontaneously tell problem-tinged stories.

As we listen to their stories of the problem, we try to put ourselves in the shoes of the people we work with. We do not assume that we understand the meaning their experience holds for them. We listen and ask. Connecting with people's experience from their perspective orients us to the specific realities that shape, and are shaped by, their personal narratives. This sort of understanding requires that we listen with focused attention, patience, and curiosity while building a relationship of mutual respect and trust.

Deconstructive listening

When we listen 'deconstructively' to people's stories, our listening is guided by the belief that those stories have many possible meanings. The meaning we as listeners make is, more often than not, at least a little different from the meaning that a speaker has intended. We seek to capitalize on this by valuing the gaps we notice in our understanding and asking people to fill in details, or by listening for ambiguities in meaning and then asking people about those ambiguities.

As people tell their stories, we reflect at intervals our sense of what they are saying and to ask whether the meaning we are making fits with their intended meaning. Even though our intention is to understand people's realities from something very close to their point of view, their realities inevitably begin to shift, at least a little, as they expand their narrative in response to our re-tellings and questions. Our very presence makes their world different. Throughout this process, we endeavour to listen with a thoughtfulness about what new constructions are emerging. We wonder aloud whether they are useful or desirable. We strive to co-create a process in which people experience choice rather than 'settled certainties' (J. Bruner, 1986) with regard to the realities that they inhabit.

Deconstructive questioning

Michael White (1991) defines deconstruction actively and politically:

> *According to my rather loose definition, deconstruction has to do with procedures that subvert taken-for-granted realities and practices: those so-called 'truths' that are split off from the conditions and the context of their production; those disembodied ways of speaking that hide their biases and prejudices; and those familiar practices of self and of relationship that are subjugating of person's lives.* (p.27)

The medical model and other discourses of modern power can lead people to a sense of themselves as 'docile bodies' (Foucault 1977), subject to knowledge and procedures in which they have no active voice. There are subjugating stories of gender, race, class, age, sexual orientation, and religion (to name a few) which are so prevalent and entrenched in our culture that we can get caught up in them without realizing it. We believe it is our responsibility as therapists to cultivate a growing awareness of the dominant (and dominating) stories in our society, and to develop ways of collaboratively examining the effects of those stories when we sense them at work in the lives and relationships of the people who consult with us.

Hare-Mustin (1994) has used the metaphor of a 'mirrored room' to talk about how the only ideas that can come up in therapy are the ideas that the people involved bring into the therapy room:

> *The therapy room is like a room lined with mirrors. It reflects back only what is voiced within it ... If the therapist and family are unaware of marginalized discourses, such as those associated with members of subordinate gender, race, and class groups, those discourses remain outside the mirrored room.* (p.22)

This notion implies that we therapists must continually reflect on the discourses that shape our perceptions of what is possible, both for ourselves and for the people we work with. Such reflection puts us in the position to ask deconstructive questions – questions whose aim is to examine problems in detail and expose discourses that support them.

Externalizing conversations

White (1987, 1988/9, 1989; see also Epston 1993) has introduced the idea that the person is not the problem, but the problem is the problem. 'Externalization' is a practice supported by the belief that a problem is something operating on or having an impact on or pervading a person's life, something separate and different from the person.

We believe that listening with the belief that problems are separate from people has a powerful deconstructive effect. It biases us to interact differently with people than we would if we saw them as intrinsically problematic. It creates a different receiving context for people's stories; one in which we can work to understand their problems without seeing the people themselves as problematic or pathological. In this kind of context, people's stories almost always become less restrictive.

We can expose dominant discourses by asking externalizing questions about contextual influences on the problem. What 'feeds' the problem? What 'starves' it? Who benefits from it? In what settings might the problematic attitude be useful? Which people would proudly advocate for the problem? What groups of people would definitely be opposed to it and its intentions? Questions such as these invite people to consider how the entire context of their lives affects the problem and vice versa.

As Reiss (1985, p.257) indicates, a family's construction of reality requires support from outside the family: 'Indeed, the family is sustained by, and contributes to, the constructions of the community in which it lives'. Many power imbalances in couples are coached and supported by power imbalances in the larger culture; imbalances that are supported by the dominant stories about class, gender, sexual orientation, race, and so on.

As problems are externalized, it becomes established that, rather than *being* the problem, the person or couple has a *relationship* with the problem. Both members of a couple have the opportunity to describe their relationships with problems in a variety of ways. One of the consequences of an externalizing conversation is that it becomes clear that both partners have relationships with the problems they name.

In externalizing conversations, we are particularly interested to hear descriptions of the effects of problems. Asking about the effects of a problem on both members of a couple, their lives, and their relationships can be particularly helpful. It helps keep the identity of the problem separate from either partner. It mobilizes the members of the couple to join together in opposing the effects of the problem. This is particularly helpful in situations in which the problem has kept them apart. People can stop thinking about themselves or their relationships as inherently problematic, and instead can consider their relationships with problems and whether they want to revise them.

Naming the problem and the project

When people name a problem, they begin the process of externalization. Naming a problem can also be a way of examining a problem and thinking differently about it. It can be poetic and compelling.

We recently saw a young heterosexual couple. The man described the problem as waking him in the middle of the night with a gun to his head. When we asked him to name the problem (which he had been referring to as 'anxiety attacks'), he called it 'the thief' because it was trying to steal his sleep. His partner, who had been scornful of the fear and difficulty sleeping until this point, could easily relate to the terror of a burglary in the dark of night. She began to appreciate her partner's bravery in facing it alone. She suggested that he wake her so that she could help.

As we ask people to evaluate their relationship to problems, we often begin to hear what they would prefer. We are especially interested in hearing about preferred directions in life. We listen for words in people's descriptions that might serve as good names for projects. We ask questions inviting them to name projects. These questions can be quite direct. For example, let's say a couple has named 'blaming' as a problem. They are recounting an incident in which they could have gotten caught up in blaming, but did not. Julie tells how she finished a major project at work, let Fran know it was finally done, and described a way she would like to celebrate. Fran did not arrange the dinner Julie would have liked that night and did not even come home until late in the evening. In the past, 'blaming' would have convinced Julie that Fran did not really care about the relationship. This time Julie was able to escape 'blaming', ask Fran what her intention was, and believe Fran's answer. In such an instance, we might ask Julie whether asking about Fran's intention instead of assuming she knew it reflected a preferred direction in life – one that blaming could have kept her from seeing. If Julie agreed, we could ask whether this direction represented a project that the couple was interested in. If they were, we could ask what name they would give the project.

Some problems and projects are shared by partners of a couple. Others are of concern to one partner, but not to the other. Witnessing each other's stories and hearing the problems and projects that shape them may be very important to a couple, even though the partners do not have a shared focus.

As the partners in a couple name problems and projects, we keep track of them. The explicit and direct discussion of projects and their contrast to problems can be a vital part of therapy. Such discussion brings forth and thickens the counterplots to problematic stories. It heightens the meaning that is made of particular experiences. Without an identified counterplot, experiences that lie outside the problem story may go unnoticed or seem trivial. With a counterplot, people can perceive shape and meaning in their non-problematic experiences. For example, once the partners in a couple have agreed on 'listening more with our hopes and less with our fears' as a shared project, any conversation they have can be plotted into the narrative of how hopes and fears influence their listening.

Until such a project is explicitly discussed and agreed upon, conversations may be given many different meanings or no meaning at all.

We keep projects present in the therapy through short names or phrases like 'growing intimacy', 'having a voice', or 'standing against violence'. These names often shift as the therapy progresses, and it is a therapist's job to keep up with the couple's changes in language and conceptualization. We seek personal, evocative, and poetic names for problems and projects. Throughout therapy, we ask questions that invite people to shape their perceptions, thoughts, feelings, and actions into stories according to the plots and counterplots they identify as meaningful for their lives.

Unique outcomes

Our entryway for inviting people to tell and live new stories is through 'unique outcomes'. A unique outcome, as noted earlier, is any event that would not have been predicted in light of a problem-saturated story. A unique outcome may be a plan, action, feeling, statement, desire, dream, thought, belief, ability, or commitment (Morgan 2000). Unique outcomes constitute openings that, through questions and reflective discussion, can be developed into new stories.

Sometimes couples offer unique outcomes quite directly. For example, someone describing a problem may say, 'It's not always like that', and go on to describe a unique outcome. It is not unusual, as couples become involved in the re-authoring process, for them to save up new unique outcomes to tell their therapist. At other times, unique outcomes are so buried in people's descriptions of their problematic stories that it is important to listen very carefully if we are not to miss them. For example, if one partner says, 'Once in a while I get through to him, but usually ...' and then proceeds to tell a problematic story, if we are listening closely, we can be curious about the 'once in a while' part, just as we would be curious about the answers to direct unique outcome questions.

Sometimes we notice events that, given the problematic story, we would not have predicted: partners who believe they have communication problems eloquently describing the problem, or one partner showing up on time to meet the other for therapy even though the problematic story is one of irresponsibility.

Most often, openings develop 'spontaneously' in ways like those we have been describing, as we listen deconstructively and ask couples about the effects of problems on their lives and relationships. If openings do not develop spontaneously, we can inquire more directly about their existence. When we are working with an externalized problem, a straightforward way of looking for openings is to ask about the influence of one or both partners on the life of the problem. That is, we ask questions such as these: 'Has there ever been a time when the problem tried to get the upper hand, but you were able to resist its influence?' or 'Have you ever been able to escape the problem for even a few minutes?' or 'Is the problem *always* with you?' When questions of this sort follow a detailed inquiry into the effects of the problem on the person or couple, people can usually find instances in which they were able to elude the problem's influence. Each such instance is a potential opening onto an alternative life narrative.

Developing stories from unique outcomes

Once we have agreed upon a preferred opening that seems relevant and interesting to one or both partners of a couple, we invite them to develop it into an alternative story. We do not have a formula to follow in this process, but we do keep in mind that stories involve events organized by plot through time in particular contexts, and that they usually include more than one person. A big part of what lets new stories make a difference in people's lives is that, in telling them to other people, a performance of meaning occurs. We work to make the therapy conversation a ritual space in which the performance of meaning can occur. Ideally, people relive the events as they tell them. We can facilitate this by asking questions to develop a story rich in detail and meaning.

White (White & Epston 1990), following Bruner (1986), speaks of the 'dual landscapes' of *action* and *consciousness* (or, in his more recent work, *identity*). He suggests that the stories constituting people's lives unfold in both these landscapes, and that it can be helpful for therapists to inquire about both. Let us look first at the landscape of action.

The landscape of action includes *detail* in *multiple modalities* involving the viewpoints of *multiple characters* in a particular *scene or setting*. It also includes the action itself. What happened, in what sequence, involving which characters?

Let us take the very simple example of Jack and Lisa at an initial therapy appointment, saying that their relationship has been deteriorating for years and that this is the first time they have sought out therapy. We might wonder whether simply deciding and following through to come to therapy is a unique outcome. The following are some questions we might ask:

- *Who actually made the suggestion that you come to therapy?*
- *What was the look on Jack's face when you suggested it? Did the look change as you talked more?*
- *Jack, what did you think when Lisa first made the suggestion? How did that change for you as you talked?*
- *Were there conversations or interactions between the two of you that prompted you to bring this up, Lisa? Was there something Jack said?*
- *Jack, do you remember that? What were you thinking that got you to say that?*
- *Who would be most pleased that you have taken this step? What would they say about it?*

In the landscape of action, we are interested in constructing an 'agentive self' with people. That is, we ask questions with an eye to enhancing those aspects of the emerging story that support 'personal agency' (Adams-Westcott, Dafforn, & Sterne 1993). The very act of re-authoring requires and demonstrates personal agency, and most people experience that in this work. We go a step further in making personal agency apparent by asking, in a variety of ways, how people have accomplished what they have.

In the example above, we might ask the following questions for this purpose:

- *Given the hopelessness you described, Lisa, what did you draw on in deciding to do something in the face of it?*
- *Were you preparing somehow to take this step? What went into that preparation?*
- *Jack, do you think that Lisa knew that you would be willing to come? How did you get past the hopelessness to agree on doing something so foreign?*

We think about the *shape* of a story as it comes forth: What happened before the unique outcome? How smoothly did things unfold? Were there false starts involved? What did this particular episode lead to? In this regard, we are especially interested to know whether there is a 'turning point', a place where the story changes for the good. Although 'turning point' is not a fitting metaphor for everyone in every situation, when it is, it distinguishes a significant event that we can plot in time. We believe it is useful to focus special attention on this sort of event, bringing forth even more shape and detail, perhaps even treating it as a story within a story.

No matter how vivid a story is in the landscape of action, if it is to have *meaning*, it must also be developed in the landscape of identity. By 'the landscape of identity', we refer to that imaginary territory in which people plot the meanings, desires, intentions, beliefs, commitments, motivations, values, and the like that relate to their experience in the landscape of action. In other words, in the landscape of identity, people reflect on the implications of experiences storied in the landscape of action.

In order to explore the landscape of identity, we ask what we (Freedman & Combs 1993) call 'meaning questions'. These are questions that invite people to step back from the landscape of action and reflect on the wishes, motivations, values, beliefs, learning, implications, and so forth that lead to and flow from the actions they have recounted. For example, we may ask:

- *What do you think it says about your relationship that you agreed to come together to therapy?*
- *Does it characterize the way the two of you do things to have secret hope in the face of hopelessness?*

In co-authoring stories, we move between the landscape of action and the landscape of identity, weaving the two back and forth again and again.

Time: Developing a 'history of the present' and extending the story into the future

White & Epston (1990) writes:

> *Social scientists became interested in the text analogy following observations that, although a piece of behavior occurs in time in such a way that it no longer exists in the present by the time it is attended to, the meaning that is inscribed into the behavior survives across time ... In striving to make sense of life, persons face the task of arranging their experiences of events in sequences across time in such a way as to arrive at a coherent account of themselves and the world around them.* (p.9)

In rendering such accounts, once a preferred event has been identified, we want to link that event to other preferred events across time; so that their meanings survive, and so that the events and their meanings can thicken a person's or couple's narrative in preferred ways. Therefore, once a preferred event is identified and storied, we ask questions to link it to other past events and develop the story of those events. Here are some examples of questions that might identify such events:

- *When you think back, what events come to mind that you might be building on that reflect other times when you could have been pulled apart, but that you came together as a couple?*
- *If we were to interview friends who have known you throughout your relationship, who might have predicted that the two of you would have been able to accomplish this? What memories might they share with us that would have led them to predict this?*

We can also ask how the emerging new story influences a person's ideas about the future. As people free more and more of their pasts from the grip of problem-dominated stories, they are able to envision, expect, and plan toward less problematic futures. We might ask:

- *We have just been talking about an accomplishment and several events in the past that paved the way for this accomplishment. If you think of these events as creating a kind of direction in your lives, what do you think will be the next step?*

- *You have learned some things about each other that have changed your view of each other and of the relationship. If you keep this new view in your hearts, how do you think the future might be different?*

Reflecting

Including time and space for reflection in therapy promotes experience of experience, and it is through the experience of reflecting on our experience that we make meaning of it. While the practice of reflection may occur even when we do not formally encourage it, such 'natural' reflection does not necessarily focus on the preferred experiences or new narratives that are developing in therapeutic conversations.

In our discussion of 'telling and witnessing', we have outlined possible reflecting structures: one partner reflecting on the other's story, the therapist reflecting, and a reflecting team or outsider witness group reflecting. In this section, we describe how we focus reflecting conversations.

Stories need listeners as well as tellers. It is through the interpersonal, societal practice of telling and re-telling of stories that they take on enough substance to change people's lives. When we ask one partner to witness the other's story, we hope that he or she will hear it in a new way. We invite reflections so that each partner can give voice to what he or she witnesses. We ask general questions such as the following:

- *What was it like to hear what Brad was saying?*
- *What thoughts were you having while Linda was talking?*

And we ask questions that more directly invite people to respond to unique outcomes and preferred directions that they might have heard in our conversation with their partners. The following are examples:

- *Were you surprised when Raoul described you as taking the time to let others know you care?*
- *What did it mean to you to hear Chantal say how important the relationship is to her?*

We then make space for the original teller to respond to his or her partner's reflections.

Whenever possible, we use reflecting teams made up of therapists (Andersen 1987), or outsider-witness groups (White 1997) made up of people asked to participate because of some type of insider knowledge to increase the audience for tellings and re-tellings. For example, if we are working with a couple struggling with infertility, we might ask other couples who have been through infertility struggles to join the group, with the couple's permission. When we have a reflecting team or an outsider-witness group we structure it in a very particular way that includes four parts (Cohen, Combs, DeLaurenti, DeLaurenti, Freedman, Larimer & Shulman 1998; White 1995).

In the first part, the therapist interviews the couple while the outsider-witness group observes the interview from behind a one-way mirror (or at a bit of a distance). In the second part, the group switches places with the couple and the therapist. The couple and therapist listen as the group members have a conversation, raising questions and commenting about what they have watched. In the third part, the couple and therapist switch back to their original places, and the couple responds to the reflections as the group observes. In the fourth part, everyone meets together for the purpose of deconstructing the interview or making it transparent. The therapist and outsider-witness group members respond to questions anyone has about their questions, purposes, and the directions they pursued in the interview.

In the second part of the interview, if an outsider-witness group or a reflecting team with little experience is reflecting, the therapist may ask questions drawing out team members, keeping the focus on what moved team members and on possible preferred directions that emerged during the interview. We ask team members to situate their reflections in their own experience, to acknowledge the trust the members of the couple are showing in opening their lives to the presence of others, and to comment on the difference bein[illegible]rt of the conversation makes to their own lives.

Documenting and circulating new stories

Because we believe that the new stories that emerge in therapy become transformative as they are enacted outside the therapy room, we are interested in documenting and circulating the new stories (White & Epston 1990). We take notes in therapy that document new stories as they develop. We often refer back to these notes and read them aloud. When couples take stands or achieve new things or reach turning points, we may create a document or certificate together that formalizes this newly distinguished event in their story. We often make videotapes for their library in which they reflect on how far they have come. We may make tapes or documents about what they have learned that can be used by others facing similar problems (White & Epston 1990). Through this kind of exchange, couples can band together with others in virtual leagues.

We sometimes write letters between therapy meetings. In these letters, we reflect on unique outcomes and ask questions that we have not asked in the therapy conversation. We hope that this will thicken and extend the knowledge that has begun to emerge there. We sometimes generate formal documents that list important elements of new narratives (Freedman & Combs 1997). To encourage the circulation of this knowledge, we invite people to share these documents with other people in their lives.

Curative factors in couple therapy/mechanisms of change

We believe that we all live our lives through stories – the stories we tell and the stories others tell about us. Those stories carry the meaning of our lives; they organize the way we experience our relationships, our identities, and the possibilities our lives hold. We think that people's experience of the meaning of their lives and relationships changes through changes in their life narratives. As their narratives change, what they do and what they perceive change as well. We facilitate this process by asking questions to highlight unstoried events, to encourage meaning making around those events, and then to tie the meaning to actions and contexts.

People's life narratives are condensations and abstractions – they contain only a small portion of the events and circumstances of their lives. Of the countless events that occur each day, only a few are storied and given meaning. When couples come to therapy, their accounts of their relationships are generally problematic and limited. This has to do, at least in part, with larger cultural stories or discourses, which support particular sets of stories and meanings and not others.

We approach therapy as an experiential process through which people reclaim, relive, and make meaning of stories that add new substance and possibilities to their lives. In our work with couples, it is also a process in which partners witness each other storying alternative events.

One of us recently had an experience with someone in therapy that illustrates the way lives change when narratives change. Rhonda, a 42-year-old woman, had been sued for malpractice some 15 years previously. Although the suit was settled out of court, there was considerable publicity and scandal. After that lawsuit, Rhonda's experience at first was that she felt devastated. As time passed, she felt numb. Her life was on hold. Although she did not find her relationship with Greg to be satisfying, she stayed in it. She stayed in her job. Life went on, but she did not. She missed the years during which she could have made the choice to have children.

After 13 years, she started therapy and began to reclaim her life. She began to consider her career and whether she would like to interview for other jobs. She ended the relationship with Greg and became involved in what she described as the best relationship of her life; with Jeff.

One day Jeff said, 'I can't believe you stayed in that relationship with Greg for so long. Why did you do it?' Rhonda said that she did not know, and they became involved in talking about other things. Two days later, Jeff apologized profusely to Rhonda, saying that he had been really thoughtless in asking that question about Greg. He had somehow forgotten about the whole lawsuit and how it had put her life on hold. Rhonda burst into gales of laughter and told him that she had forgotten too!

She, of course, knew that it had happened, but it was no longer the central story of her life. Other stories had been told, retold, witnessed, documented, and, more importantly, re-experienced. The thicker version of Rhonda's narrative supported new actions and possibilities: a new relationship, new ways of thinking about work, and many smaller changes. The way Rhonda experienced her life had changed through a re-storying of events. Her immersion in the alternative stories supported new relationships and other possibilities.

Another way of describing our ideas about change is to say that in successful therapy new meanings are performed. 'Performance of meaning' is a concept that narrative therapists have borrowed from poststructural anthropology, particularly from the work of Barbara Myerhoff (1982, 1986), who gave numerous examples of how, instead of being an innate quality, meaning arises through performance. Unless a story is told and re-told; circulated, written down, acted out, sung, etc., it has no lasting meaning. In the light of this notion, the new strands of story that emerge in response to our questions must be circulated and put into action before they can become meaningful.

When Jeff apologized to Rhonda for his memory lapse, he was performing meaning around the lapse. When Rhonda realized that she too had lost track of those 13 painful years, she added another layer of meaning to Jeff's. Rhonda's re-telling of the incident in therapy was a big performance of meaning, and in that performance, her new, joyous relationship with Jeff became appreciably more real and memorable.

We believe that change occurs through the performance of meaning that takes place in waves of telling and re-telling such as these.

Treatment applicability

For us, the most important aspect of narrative therapy is the worldview. Narrative practices flow from a narrative/poststructuralist worldview. Once we begin to see problems as separate from people and to situate problems in socio-cultural discourses, we no longer see people in ways that support making traditional, expert, individual diagnoses. Once we enter into ideas that support collaboration, we no longer experience ourselves as the possessors of expert knowledge about what would be most helpful to people. Instead, we begin to appreciate the insider knowledge that people acquire through struggling with particular problems in particular contexts. The narrative worldview leads to a shift in perception. We do not stand outside our work and assess it by scientific criteria. Instead, we ask people in an ongoing way whether the therapy is helpful and how it is helpful.

If a member of a couple wonders whether medication might be helpful, or requests a formal assessment of a particular problem, we talk about it and, if the couple chooses, we make a referral to someone who might collaboratively facilitate a decision about medication, diagnosis, or the like. We do not consider medication or testing a part of narrative therapy, but we support people in exploring whatever kind of approach they think might be helpful.

We have found that the narrative approach has general applicability. Although the length, intensity, and specific outcome of therapy vary from problem to problem and from context to context, the approach is as effective for couples seeking pre-marital counseling as it is for couples struggling to reclaim their relationship from violence and abuse.

However, our experience is that some couples prefer a different kind of therapy relationship than we offer. Some people are seeking instruction or expert advice. Others are more interested in exploring their past histories to 'find out' why they are in the situations they find themselves in. We ask people regularly how the therapy is going for them, and we are open and willing to refer couples if they are seeking a different kind of therapy relationship.

At the same time, we have discovered that most couples coming to therapy are not as concerned about how the therapy relationship is structured as they are about whether their relationship improves. Because popular notions of therapy include descriptions such as 'getting to the root of the problem', they may initially use words that would seem to indicate a preference for a different kind of therapy relationship. With further conversation, we have found that most couples are simply interested in improving their relationships.

Case illustration

> *Since one of us (JF) was the therapist working with Mark and Victoria, we have written this section primarily in her voice, from her point of view. Throughout the description of the therapy we have also offered commentary in italics to help readers relate the clinical illustration to the first part of this chapter.*

Victoria was referred by a colleague of mine who was her neighbor. On the phone, she told me that she and her husband had been experiencing problems for some time and that they couldn't work them out on their own.

We usually begin therapy with a new couple by getting to know each member before we get to know the problem. Otherwise, the problem might color our view of them and keep us from seeing possibilities for them outside of the problem. We hope that starting this way helps people feel free to talk about aspects of their relationship and experience that they like, not just those that are problematic.

Since I had spoken with Victoria on the phone, I began the meeting by talking with Mark. He told me that he was 41 years old and that he lived in a small city in Wisconsin, about an hour and a half away, where he held a job as a supervisor in a manufacturing plant. He had an 18-year-old daughter by a previous marriage, whom he did not see as often as he would like. She seemed to initiate visits only when she wanted money. Mark had been divorced for 13 years and married to Victoria for 8. He enjoyed playing cards, riding a motorcycle, and doing projects around his house.

Victoria told me that she was 40 years old, an artist, and a professor in a fine arts program. She loved going to galleries, seeing films and traveling. For the last three years, because of her work teaching, she had lived separately from Mark, who had to stay in Wisconsin for his work. Before Victoria found her teaching post, the couple had lived together in Wisconsin.

The tone of this early part of the interview was highly interactive. Jill did not listen to what Mark and Victoria said as bits of 'information' that she could use to form an assessment. Instead, she was interested in getting to know them as people. She also wanted to present herself as a person, rather than as a representative of professional expertise. She hoped this would contribute to reducing the hierarchy and establishing a collaborative relationship.

After hearing a bit from the couple, I asked whether they would like to ask me any questions.

Jill's intention in asking was to undermine the hierarchy a bit and to create an opportunity for transparency. We want couples to know that we will welcome their questions throughout therapy.

Mark had no questions right then, but Victoria was interested in knowing what I liked to read. We talked a few minutes about books and authors.

We are interested in creating a context in which people's stories can be spoken and heard. In our experience, by the time couples get to therapy, the interweaving stories of their problems tend to follow a well-rehearsed choreography. Blame and defensiveness often overshadow any hopes and constructive intentions either party has for the relationship. We want to facilitate something different from the outset. For that purpose, during much of the therapy (this varies for different couples) we speak to one person at a time, with the other partner in the position of witnessing his or her story. As we have previously described, at particular points we turn to the partner and ask for reflections. Sometimes we explain the structure, saying something like this: 'I am going to talk with Mark for a few minutes and ask you to just listen. After we talk for a bit, you'll get a chance to respond to what you've heard. Then we'll switch and I'll talk with you for a while. Will that be OK?' If either partner seems dubious or uncertain about this idea, we will explain that when one person describes an irksome or scary difficulty, the other often feels put on the spot to point out mistakes or counter with a different description. Rather than really listening to the partner's story, the listener composes a rebuttal while the partner is talking. We would like to offer a context where people can really hear their partners, knowing that each person will have an opportunity to tell his or her story and have it heard.

Once we know a bit about each partner, we want to hear and understand the couple's stories of what is problematic. We collaborate with the couple in naming the problem or problems and ask questions to begin deconstructing those problems. We also listen for openings to new, preferred stories.

Jill began a discussion of the problem with Mark because of her awareness that women often bear responsibility for the wellbeing of relationships. Since Victoria had made the appointment and was most active in the early conversation, Jill wanted to offer Mark the possibility of taking active responsibility for the well-being of the relationship.

I moved into a witnessing structure casually, simply speaking directly to Mark and making eye contact primarily with him while Victoria listened. I asked Mark to tell me about what brought the couple to therapy. He spoke rather hesitantly about 'things deteriorating': Victoria was coming home to Wisconsin less, and he was coming to Chicago more; she was always wanting to talk, and he was quiet; she was curious and motivated, and he was trying to be more active and enthusiastic but feeling as if he never quite made it. I wondered what the effects of these differences were. *('Differences' was the name Jill heard Mark using for what was problematic.)* In our ensuing discussion he created a list of effects: frustration, anger, and defensiveness, which got him to 'clam up'.

When I asked Victoria what she was thinking while Mark talked *(notice the beginning of the telling and reflecting rhythm)*, she said that she had been unhappy for a couple of years, but she hadn't realized that he had been too. In response to my questions inviting her evaluation, she said that this was good to realize because at least they were together in their experience.

Later in the conversation, Victoria said that she felt as if she had been marking time. She declared that she wanted someone to go forward with her to share knowledge and challenge her – somebody who knew things she did not and could open doors for her. She ended by stating, 'This relationship has been the safe harbor, but I want a shift to rockier waters'.

In Mark's reflections, he said that he could understand how Victoria valued excitement. He said that he valued it too. What was important for him was to share both exciting and quiet times with someone else, and to be with someone who enjoyed the same things he did. When I asked how much of that he already got from this relationship, he said 50-60%. He wondered whether it might help their relationship if, instead of relying on each other, they each found friends to join them in activities that did not interest the other.

Victoria broke into the conversation and wailed, 'What can we be intimate about, then?'

As the conversation continued, they tentatively agreed on naming the problems 'distance' and 'frustration'. *(In this instance, Mark and Victoria named shared problems. In other situations, each partner may name a different problem. We do not want people to name shared problems unless that fits their experience.)* Over the remainder of the first interview, and during the second, we mapped the effects of distance and frustration.

For Victoria, although she had not experienced herself as looking for other men, the distance and frustration had contributed to what she called 'two and a half relationships' with other men. The half relationship involved frequent meetings and conversations, but was not sexual, as the other two had been. Distance had given her room to see Mark in a different, less favorable light and to have more independent dreams. Seeing him in this new light led her to decide that she did not respect some things about him: he did not have 'enough' education, he did not discuss things enough, and reading was a chore for him. Seeing Mark in this way created turmoil for Victoria. She could no longer see the relationship fitting with her larger goals, and she worried that Mark was no longer getting enough from it either.

Mark also agreed that distance and frustration had led Victoria to become involved in other relationships and contributed to their relationship 'breaking down'. When we unpacked what Mark meant by the relationship 'breaking down', we came up with this list:

- mistrust and anger,
- impatience and sometimes disgust on Victoria's part when they were together,
- Mark's experience of not being able to do anything right.

The effects of distance and frustration were taking a toll on Mark's and Victoria's relationships with themselves. Victoria felt horrible both about the pain she was causing Mark and about how she was not always being honest with herself. Mark found himself more and more involved with self-degradation.

Once we had unpacked some of the effects of distance and frustration, I asked about the partners' evaluation of these effects. I wondered whether they wanted to continue in their current relationship with the effects. I asked questions about each effect, such as: 'What is it like to be subjected to self-degradation? Is turmoil something that you want for your life. Why or why not?'

Early in this process, Mark suggested that some background information might be helpful. He told me that when he and Victoria married, they vowed to give each other room to grow and promised to help each other. He had reminded himself of this when Victoria first became interested in another man. For him, the problem was not other relationships per se, but the fact that he felt pushed away while they were going on. Mistrust and anger were problematic, he said, because he would like Victoria and himself to be easy with each other and to be friends again. He could be OK with the amount of time apart if he felt respected, appreciated, cared about, and connected. He did not want disgust and self-degradation to influence his life and relationship. In fact, Mark took a firm stand against disgust and self-degradation, saying that he would like to be together with Victoria, but not if that meant he also had to live with disgust and self-degradation.

When her turn came, Victoria said that the lack of respect she experienced in relation to Mark was not something that she wanted. It created turmoil in her life, and what she wanted instead was to be at peace in the relationship. She did not want peace at any cost. She wanted to step out and be bigger in what she did and what she dreamed. She thought that some of the impatience had to do with not knowing how to step out. As she considered it more, she realized that the impatience did not really serve her well. She thought that there was room to include Mark in her dreams and she realized that impatience stood in the way of that. She said that she would like to talk with Mark about how he might be included in her dreams.

I made note of her wish and of Mark's 50-60% satisfaction. They were potential unique outcomes that I wanted to come back to and ask more about, but first I asked about lack of respect and how it influenced Victoria's experience of Mark. She had mentioned 'things about him' (not having a college education, not discussing things as much as she would like, and finding reading a chore) as contributing to the lack of respect. I asked what those things meant to her, and Victoria said: 'The first thing that came to mind was that he is not very intelligent, but I know he is intelligent'. When I asked how she knew he was intelligent, she described how Mark had advised her in setting up her studio and creating a marketing plan for her work. He did not simply encourage her; he had challenged her in ways that had been quite helpful. She credited him with much of the success she had experienced in the business aspect of her work. She appreciated how intelligently he helped her map out a plan. He did not make assumptions, was very deliberate in setting things in order, and came up with creative ideas.

In the following conversation, Jill asked questions that helped Victoria unmask some of the discourses that tricked her into a problematic view of Mark.

I wondered, given everything she had just said, how Victoria could have been tricked into doubting Mark's intelligence. She thought it odd as well. When I asked who might think that not having a college education, not discussing things, and not enjoying reading indicated a lack of intelligence, she began to wonder about how teaching in a university had influenced her. We talked about different values in the university and in what Victoria called 'the everyday world'. She said that this discussion really clarified some things for her. When she and Mark first got together, she was not part of the university. She was an artist barely making it in a little town in Wisconsin. And in her situation there, she had not experienced the same feelings about Mark's education and reading habits.

When I turned to him, Mark agreed that things had been different when Victoria lived in Wisconsin. He added that the feelings of disgust seemed to be most apparent after going to the movies. Victoria and her Chicago friends had a way of discussing movies that was not meaningful to Mark. He did not understand why discussing movies seemed so important to Victoria. He now wondered if this discussion thing was part of the university environment. *(Mark was now tracing the feelings of disgust to 'the university environment', not to himself or Victoria.)*

Victoria nodded in agreement, but added that she enjoyed the process of critique. Just as she was beginning to declare that she did not want the university dictating her perceptions, Mark interrupted.

'You know I'm going to college', he said. I learned that, at Victoria's suggestion, he had decided to pursue labor studies. What Victoria did not know until now was that he was enjoying it. 'I like being opened up and seeing new things and meeting new people', he said.

When I asked Victoria what it was like to hear about Mark's experience, she said that she felt better just knowing about it. She also appreciated the way he was standing up for himself. 'It is pretty intelligent!' she said.

I asked whether Mark's going to college meant that he, too, would take on university values. Mark said that he preferred to have his own values. Victoria agreed, saying that his approach to school was one she could respect.

In the first two meetings, Jill asked questions that helped Victoria and Mark name and map the effects of some of the problems that were undermining their relationship. Victoria and Mark evaluated the problems and stated their preferences for how to relate to the problems. Jill's questions helped Mark and Victoria expose the role that social class (in the form of 'university values') played in shaping the meanings they had made about some of their differences. Several unique outcomes – things that would not be predicted by the problematic story – had come to light, but Jill, Mark, and Victoria had not yet developed a story to support any of these.

At our third meeting, because colleagues were visiting from out of town, we were able to have a reflecting team. When I asked Victoria and Mark, they were open to the experience and also gave permission to make a videotape that they could keep to review later.

After Victoria and Mark had been introduced to the team members, I approached the conversation with curiosity about whether any of the unique outcomes I had previously noted had captured their imaginations. I started the interview by reading my notes aloud, reviewing our conversations, and asking how things had gone since we last met.

Victoria said that she had been thinking about dreams since the last meeting. She had mentioned her dreams the last time and wondered how Mark would fit into them, but what she had realized since our conversation was that she did not know what his dreams were. She wanted to hear his dreams.

Mark was reluctant to talk about his dreams. When I asked questions to unpack his reluctance, he named fear and insecurity as problems, saying they kept him from being able to hold his own in what he called 'these kinds of discussions that Victoria always wants to have'. As we talked more, he said that he just did not have the dreams of huge accomplishment and artistic achievement that Victoria did. Instead, he looked forward to each weekend when he would do something like make shelves for the family room. After he described the differences a bit more, I referred back to our conversation about the difference in university values and everyday values. I wondered whether this was another example of that difference. He thought it was. I asked what he thought the difference talked him into. 'Insecurity', he said. 'Defensiveness'.

Just as I was about to ask questions about the effects of fear, insecurity, and defensiveness, Mark told me that things are not always that way. He began to describe an experience he had at fantasy baseball camp. I had never heard of fantasy baseball camp, so I asked him to tell me about it. He explained that fantasy baseball camp was a place where, for a fee, ordinary guys could spend a week playing baseball with major league players in a major league stadium.

Victoria had accompanied Mark on his week in the big leagues. She described seeing his skin glow and his eyes shine as he savored playing and trying to accomplish something. They spent the greater part of the hour reliving detailed stories of that time, in which fear and insecurity could have stopped him, but instead he triumphed. For Victoria, remembering these experiences was 'fantastic'. I asked when else she had appreciated and enjoyed Mark the way she did at fantasy baseball camp. She told me about a camping trip they had gone on with his daughter, early in their relationship. Everything had gone wrong. Victoria found herself burrowing miserably into the tent, shrinking from the rain and mud puddles outside, and wishing she were anywhere but there. Then Mark began dancing and singing in the rain with Emily, his daughter. He kept calling out to Victoria until she joined them. This was now her most treasured memory of camping.

I asked whether it was more important for Mark to stay in touch with this version of himself or for Victoria to be in touch with it. It turned out that it was important for both of them. For Victoria, it meant that she could take Mark to a cocktail party or a movie with her colleagues without worrying that he would have nothing to contribute. It helped her see how he could fit in; it even reminded her of times in the past when he had already fit in. She described two incidents that the 'university values' (*classism-tinged*) perception of Mark had kept her from remembering. For Mark, the 'fantasy baseball camp' version of himself meant he could 'keep on keeping on' instead of getting bogged down in insecurity.

When we switched places, the team members reflected on different aspects of the conversation. Here I summarize only the comments that Mark and Victoria chose to respond to. One team member noted that Mark said he did not know how to talk about his dreams, yet he brought up fantasy baseball camp. She couldn't imagine a more vivid way to talk about dreams. Another member wondered how someone who only had small dreams was able to make such a grand dream – fantasy baseball camp – come true. A third comment had to do with singing and dancing in the rain. The team member who commented wondered if that event had to do with Mark's not allowing his dreams to get rained out.

Mark and Victoria were moved by the comments of the reflecting team. They came back into the room and told more stories about fantasy baseball camp and how Mark had decided to go there. If 'university values' was the problem, I wondered, would 'dreams' have something to do with a project they could pursue in the face of that problem? They said it would, and named the project 'living our dreams'.

Victoria thought back again to the camping experience and realized that Mark had actively coaxed her out of the tent so that she could join in. She thought she had not yet done as much to pave the way for him. Victoria ended by saying that it was more usual for her to be the center of attention. The team had talked about Mark for the most part. She wondered if this was a sign that he was coming forward and growing. 'That would certainly have to do with my dream', she said.

In this interview, Mark and Victoria named a project. They began developing an alternative story and a 'history of the present'. Fortuitously, this new story had a reflecting audience of several people, and it was documented on videotape.

The 'fantasy baseball camp' interview seemed to be a turning point in the relationship. Victoria opened the fourth meeting by talking about the 'new Mark' who now clearly cared about the relationship. She described him as being more inquisitive and outgoing.

When I turned to Mark, he said that he experienced himself as a better listener. He thought that others around him noticed the change as well. They almost had to have noticed, because he had been speaking his thoughts aloud. He was surprised to discover that sharing his thoughts made him feel better. He said that these changes were possible because he realized he had something to say and to contribute. As we developed the story of this realization, Mark began to wonder whether the reflecting team had helped him reach it. He spoke about how moving it was to feel appreciated by strangers who heard him talking about his life. Through their eyes, he had a greater appreciation of himself. Just realizing that he could make a contribution made him more aware of what went on around him. He now knew that he had abilities to do lots of things.

We have heard this kind of response to a reflecting team many times. These responses inspire us to work in teams whenever we can.

After drawing Mark out about the meaning of the new events, I turned to Victoria who had been witnessing the elaboration of the new story. When I asked her what stood out in my conversation with Mark, she said that she always knew Mark had this in him. While he was speaking, she kept remembering examples of his enthusiasm for doing new things. She thought they had been stuck for a long time on a plateau, but now they were climbing the next mountain.

The usefulness of the reflecting position stands out here. In hearing Mark speak to Jill, Victoria reviewed the past, remembering other times that fit her view of 'the new Mark'. As Mark heard Victoria proclaim their progress as a couple, it couldn't help taking on substance. The stories of the new Mark became more real, more solid, and more memorable. Jill now asked some questions with the intention of helping the new stories continue to grow.

Mark said that it would support his reclaimed view of himself to associate with people more, whether Victoria was there or not. He was learning that he was a stronger person, but even for a strong person, being alone can foster insecurity.

I referred back to the beginning of the conversation and said to Victoria that she had named the changes we were discussing 'the new Mark'. I did not want to discount Mark's changes, but I did notice that at least some of what she was calling 'new' had strong roots in the past. I asked whether the new Mark had something to do with 'the new Victoria' or 'the new relationship'.

Victoria nodded and said that she had changed the way she was looking at things, and that doing so made for different possibilities in their relationship. She was now seeing beyond university values.

I wondered if during the times Victoria was in Chicago teaching, surrounded by the academic community, university values might take over again and persuade her that Mark did not fit her dreams. Victoria could see how that might be possible, so she decided to make more of an effort to include Mark in her life in the city – both in terms of inviting friends and colleagues to be with them when he was there, and talking more with him about her activities and interests at the university. Part of living their dreams for Victoria had to do with including Mark more in her life.

Mark thought he could go along with Victoria's vision, but he warned that it would be important for her to be more part of his life in Wisconsin as well.

Between meetings, during a weekend in Wisconsin, Victoria asked Mark to read a short story she had written. Writing was not her usual medium for art, so she thought that she might be more open to Mark's ideas than she would have been with much of her art. He returned the short story to her by fax, two days after she left, having corrected the grammar.

Victoria recounted this incident during the fifth therapy meeting. She hadn't talked with Mark about her reaction to his corrections, because it seemed so closely related to what they were working on in therapy that she thought it best to wait. I asked her if her reaction would be different, depending on whether it came from university values or from living their dreams. She closed her eyes, took a deep breath, and said that yes, it was different. I asked her which reaction she preferred. She chose the one that came from including Mark in her dreams. *(Note the change in language from 'living their dreams' to 'including Mark more in her dreams'. We find that people name their problems and projects fluidly. It is important for therapists to flow along with them.)* If she kept that desire in her heart, the corrections meant that he was interested in what she did and had found a way he could contribute comfortably. I asked if there might have been other times when Mark's response to Victoria's art would have had different meaning if she had focused on her desire to include Mark in her dreams. She told three stories of incidents that now looked different. One of them had to do with a show of her work. Mark walked through the gallery with her, naming his thoughts about what the models had been for each piece. Victoria now saw that Mark was naming her inspirations and finding connections between their life and her work. University values had created an expectation of a more intellectual critique, which had kept her from seeing Mark's loving intentions at the time.

When I asked Mark what it was like to hear what Victoria saw when she followed the desire to include him in her dreams, he said it was a tremendous relief. In the past, he had felt tested when she asked him to look at her work or even to talk about a movie. He thought there was a right answer that she knew and he did not. This difference put them on unequal footing, as though she was the tester and he the student. The effect of this experience was that he felt cornered. Knowing that he did not know the right answer, his first response was to give no answer, this inevitably led to frustration for Victoria, which in turn increased his feeling of being trapped. I asked him what was different now. He said that if Victoria suspended the university values in favor of including him in her dreams, then there would not be a right answer; anything he said would mean that he was participating in her life.

Victoria agreed and said that she felt hopeful.

Mark said that this turn of events would lessen his fear. He said he already was feeling less frightened at work, and described an incident in which he stood up for himself because he was tired of being pushed around.

For Victoria, the incident at work showed that Mark was trusting his intelligence and his intuition. She saw him showing increased confidence, and she thought that as this continued it would help her know how much he had to contribute. She said that she was proud and happy that Mark was examining his life and taking some stands. She was distressed by the tester–student analogy. I asked whether she could understand where it came from. She could, and was wondering if she had invested more of herself in university values than in art. She preferred art and thought that keeping Mark more present in her art and life would help keep the balance the way she wanted it.

In this interview, power relations and class discourses were exposed in a very down-to-earth and relevant way. The metaphors of unequal footing and the tester–student relationship emerged from the conversation and contributed to the deconstruction of university values. These ideas were not introduced by Jill, but Victoria and Mark had not made these distinctions until Jill asked questions to locate their problems in the discourses of their local cultures. Through this deconstruction, Victoria and Mark were able to see possibilities that they could not see before. These possibilities offered new choices and paved the way for them to re-author their relationship, instead of allowing class differences to write its story.

At the sixth meeting, Mark and Victoria both described important ways that the relationship had moved forward. The two had talked more collaboratively about Victoria's work. They agreed that they had truly exchanged opinions. They had negotiated resolutions to disagreements without anger. Mark had brought a more positive attitude about himself to this, less influenced by fear and self-degradation. The new attitude allowed him to put his opinions forward strongly, without fear, and to listen non-defensively to Victoria's responses. He also had initiated some of their conversations, which was a new role for him. Victoria had put a whole different attitude and way of listening into practice – one that was more open and not predicated on her assumed greater knowledge in a tester–student relationship. Through reflecting on these interactions, Mark recognized that Victoria was not invested in controlling the relationship. Knowing this, he could participate with lightheartedness. For both of them, these conversations were providing more comfort about talking together. This comfort was not a new thing, but an old way of being that had slipped away from them. Near the end of the sixth meeting, in response to my questions, Victoria and Mark told some stories about past times, early in the relationship, when they had experienced the kind of comfort that they were now reclaiming.

They agreed that they were hopeful and said that it felt as though they were getting to know each other all over again. For Victoria, the next step would be to connect more emotionally and have more intimacy.

The sixth interview served to thicken Mark and Victoria's story, adding distinctions and events that contributed to an alternative narrative. The stories of past times enriched and revivified the history of the present, and Jill's final questions about next steps invited Victoria to extend the story into the near future.

Mark started the seventh meeting by saying that he was angry about Victoria's other relationships. I said that I was pulled in two different directions. The first was to respond to the anger about the relationships, but I was also intrigued by how Mark had taken the step of initiating a subject for therapy. This was something new, and I wondered whether it was a step away from fear and toward something Mark preferred. I asked Mark which of those two directions he thought was most important to address.

Here, Jill was expanding possibilities while leaving the power of choice in Mark's hands.

Mark answered, 'I guess both'. He went on to explain that although he had known about the relationships while they were occurring he had not expressed anger about them until the past weekend. Talking about anger, he said, was a step away from fear. It had been important for him to discover that talking – even about anger – helped a lot. He could be mad, express it, and maybe let go of it, and he and Victoria could stay connected.

Victoria agreed, saying that these steps were both good and scary.

I asked whether they wanted to talk more about the relationships, and both Victoria and Mark said they did not. Victoria said that the other relationships had to do with how disconnected she and Mark were. In this work, they were choosing each other again. Given this choice, there would not be other relationships.

Mark nodded. Their eyes locked.

After a pause, Victoria said that they had been spending their weekends together, but not in isolation. As a couple, they had socialized quite a bit with other people. It seemed that they were joining their lives back together.

In my prelude to the next question, I voiced a thought: 'So you are joining your lives back together ...' Victoria interrupted, 'Except in the areas of sexuality and sensuality'. She went on to explain that some months before I met them she had called a halt during sex with Mark because she felt it had no spirituality or intimacy. Mark experienced this as a rejection, and had completely removed himself sexually, believing that this was what Victoria wanted. Now there was no touching at all – no holding hands, no hugging, nothing.

I wondered if Mark's putting fear aside to voice his anger about the other relationships had something to do with Victoria bringing up their sexual relationship now, or whether it had to do with something else.

Victoria said that it had to do with joining their lives back together.

I asked if that phrase – 'joining their lives back together' – was a project they were working on with me.

They both nodded. Victoria said that joining their lives back together was a huge part of living their dreams. Mark agreed.

Victoria said that she was interested in having a sexual relationship with Mark, but also scared because so much was going well and she did not know whether this would go well.

Although I was interested in finding out about the fear, the hour was nearly over, so I did not ask about it. Instead, I wrote it down with a question mark beside it in my notes.

Mark suggested that he would be most comfortable if they approached sex as an exploration, and said that if they were going to take it on he wanted ongoing feedback.

We talked about how Victoria had been the one wanting feedback about her work, and I wondered whether they had learned anything in the process of finding a way to talk together about Mark's responses to art that might be helpful here. They agreed that assumptions and thinking there was one right way could mean trouble, and that keeping talking would make them be connected.

I asked Mark if it was important to talk more about the other relationships Victoria had been involved in the next time we met. He said that hearing that she wanted to be sexually involved with him was the important thing.

Although I expected that we would be talking about sex at the eighth meeting, Victoria and Mark talked about talking. After the seventh meeting, Mark had told Victoria how painful her sexual and romantic intimacy with other people had been for him. They told me about some of the details of the conversation. I asked them about its meaning and effects. For Mark, the conversation meant that there was growing honesty between them. For Victoria, it meant that and more. She felt that Mark had opened his experience to her so clearly that she could feel it. She said that she was happy that he had been talking more, but this was a whole different step. Mark said that Victoria had contributed to this different kind of conversation by talking more calmly and with less animosity. She said that what had changed her behavior was that she was really trying to listen to what Mark was saying. She expected this would make it possible to feel Mark's feelings as well as her own the next time she had the possibility of being with another man. But now that she and Mark were talking together, that possibility seemed very remote.

For Mark, Victoria's reaction to their conversation was quite startling. Even as he found himself initiating the conversation about her other lovers, he thought it was a mistake; surely Victoria would either think he was wrong or decide he was whining. Instead, she seemed fascinated. She told him that she just wanted to be in on what he was thinking and feeling. She said that she wanted that in all of their discussions. Mark had thought that new ideas were the only things worth contributing, and he often did not have big, shiny new ideas. He felt the fear evaporate as Victoria reiterated the importance of being included in his thoughts and feelings.

I asked Mark and Victoria about whether they each had experienced friendships in which they had felt free to say what they were thinking and feeling. Both had. Mark told about breakfasts with a roommate he had before meeting Victoria. They would sit at the kitchen table, newspapers propped in front of them, and say whatever came to mind. Mark had often been surprised when Louis referred to things he said and seemed to be affected by them. Reviewing that relationship helped Mark appreciate that he did not have to create something new to say to have something to offer. Victoria told about her best friend, Sally, whom she talked with almost every day in person or on the phone. That relationship reminded her of how precious it could be to share the details of another's life. She recognized how far away that type of sharing is from a university critique.

I wondered if we were talking about intimacy.

An important part of a therapist's job is to ask questions to slow things down, develop detail, and reflect on meaning. In Jill's report, she has omitted many of the careful, detailed questions she asked to bring forth the rich story that Mark and Victoria were telling. I (GC) hope that readers, upon reflection, can appreciate how things might have turned out quite differently without Jill's questions.

Mark and Victoria came to the ninth meeting talking about how good things had felt lately. They agreed that they were 'on the same side of the table'. They described how they were interacting together more and enjoying it. They told me that Mark had been looking at Victoria with tenderness, and Victoria had been open to that. Victoria said that she thought Mark was opening himself to her as he never had before. Mark thought that he had been just as open before, but this time Victoria was recognizing it. To Mark, that meant that she was trying and that she cared. Mark said that it was easier for him to be open because Victoria had been relaxed, approachable, and receptive. For the first time in a long time, she had told him that she loved him.

There had been more affection, including hugging each other and holding hands in public. For Mark, that meant there was more effort. For Victoria, the hugging and holding hands were outward acknowledgments of the changes under way in their relationship.

They said that the most momentous thing that they had done was make love. They were both glad to have taken that step and both thought that the most important thing was just that they did it. It signified their renewed commitment and growing love. Victoria reiterated that they had a new connection that she did not want to discount, but she felt that the lovemaking was an old routine. She felt disappointment that she hadn't taken a more active role in changing the routine. She saw that she could have added playfulness and wished that she had. She wanted to be able to communicate about their lovemaking both in and out of bed. I wondered whether anything they had learned about communicating would be helpful. 'To say what is in our hearts', she said. Mark agreed.

Once a new story begins to take on life and momentum, therapy conversations tend to be a bit looser. Without prompting, people often talk in more detail about new developments. Problems are mentioned less and less. With Mark and Victoria, Jill was still active in asking questions to draw out detail, complexity, and meaning, but there was more spontaneous talk, and the old problems were not in control of what was being said and felt.

Victoria came into the 10th meeting glowing. A week before, she had awakened in the middle of the night with severe nausea and intestinal cramping. She had called Mark, and he had jumped out of bed and driven to Chicago. A number of things were remarkable about this event, starting with Victoria's making the call. When she woke up uncomfortable and frightened, she immediately called Mark; in the past she would probably have called Sally and then they might have called a doctor or gone straight to the emergency room without even letting Mark know. The way Victoria immediately reached for the phone to dial Mark showed what a central position he now had in her life. It spoke clearly of the trust and confidence she felt for him and for their relationship. Upon answering the call, Mark was immediately reassuring and emotionally available. He offered to call a doctor or to help in any other way, all the while dressing for the ride. He never once even mentioned his commitments for the next day.

This incident was clearly meaningful for both Mark and Victoria. Jill chose to ask lots of questions to develop an ever thicker, more meaningful experience of the incident for both partners. In reflecting on this choice, we can see that it might have been useful to slow down the conversation and make sure that Jill wasn't being overly influenced by the discourse privileging couples' relationships over other kinds of relationship – especially since Mark had suggested earlier that perhaps he and Victoria should rely on people outside the relationship for some particular interests and activities. We are not separate from our culture, and we can never be aware of all the discourses that it might be helpful to deconstruct – but that doesn't mean that we shouldn't keep trying.

I reminded the partners that when they first came to see me they had named the problems they were struggling with 'distance' and 'frustration'. I wondered what this event showed about how far they had come. 'This was just the opposite!' Victoria said.

In fact, the incident meant so much to Victoria that she took another step forward emotionally. The following weekend in Wisconsin, with Mark, she went for motorcycle rides, picked apples at an orchard, and went to a birthday bash for a relative at Mark's mother's house. She could participate wholeheartedly in these events because she felt more open and trusting. She wanted to do things so that Mark could have his dreams. Before, she would have brought work with her to Wisconsin and would have spent at least part of the time holed up with it. This time, she found a way to get her work done before going.

Until Victoria described her intentions for the past weekend, Mark had not recognized the significance of the events. He had thought she just had more time. Now that he heard what the weekend had meant for Victoria, he felt less peripheral and more important in her life. For him, feeling this way was like a door opening to their future. Seeing the door made him more willing to plan their future together.

Thinking back again to our first meeting, I reminded them that Mark had said then that he got about 50-60% of what he wanted from the relationship. I wondered what they would each say now. They both said that they were at 80-85% and named the following as making the difference:

- their new way of talking,
- trust,
- each letting the other in to his or her,
- touching each other again.

What I probably would have asked if there had been more time at the 10th meeting was what Victoria and Mark could do in relation to the 15-20% of what they wanted that they were not yet getting in the relationship. They seemed to have brought the answer with them to the 11th meeting. They came in clearly focused on the 15-20%. Victoria talked about sadness and anger that had been stirred up by their sexual relationship. Mark talked about frustration and anger. Victoria said that she wanted Mark to take more authority and responsibility. Mark said that when he did, she backed away. Victoria said that there was just no context for sex. She thought things would go better if he were to stroke her hair and call her beautiful and look into her eyes as they moved into sex. Mark said, 'Why don't you just give me a script?'

As mutual blame began to take over the conversation, I asked if it would be alright if I slowed things down.

Aspects of the old, problematic story were beginning begun to influence Mark and Victoria again. This is not at all uncommon. Jill became more active in shaping the conversation, moving back into a more deliberate pattern of speaking at length with one partner before asking the other to reflect on what he or she had just heard.

After hearing a bit more of a description of their current problems, I asked whether Mark or Victoria could remember sexual experiences with each other that they felt good about. They could, but were surprised to learn that they remembered different experiences. Mark described experiences in which 'things went smoothly', he felt in charge, Victoria seemed receptive and excited throughout, and they both had orgasms. Victoria described experiences in which she felt beautiful and light.

I asked Victoria about this a bit more, and she said that probably the biggest factor for her in how well sex went was how attractive she felt. If she felt fat and sloppy, it put a damper on her participation. When she felt beautiful, which was a struggle, she could really be involved sexually. I wondered if she thought that her ideas about sex had to do with how she was brought up as a girl and a woman. She nodded and said she thought that men did worry about how they looked, but not nearly as much as women, and probably not during sex. I asked where she thought the idea of having to look a certain way came from.

'Everywhere', she said. 'Films, books, ads even ...' I asked if the images in films, books, and ads were real, and she said that they were in that they were based on real people. I mentioned that I had once worked with a woman who was a professional model. I asked whether Victoria was interested in what the model had told me about magazine covers and the like. When Victoria said she was, I told her the model had said that the people in ads were a very small percentage of real people who were being photographed at a particular age that would not last. Those people had been freshly made up and positioned in a particular way to create a particular impression. Furthermore, the final image was often airbrushed to 'improve' it even more.

Readers may see Jill as imposing her own knowledge here. To us, it is important that Jill asked Victoria if she wanted to hear her, and it is even more important that Jill was passing along local knowledge from a particular person, not disembodied expert advice.

I wondered what effect the contrived images had on Victoria. 'I'm always comparing myself', she said. 'Not favorably'. I asked if those images talked her into anything about her worth. She said that sexually she did not have much. I wondered if it really fit with her (sexually or any other way) to have her worth depend on matching an image, while leaving the expression of love, passion, creativity, playfulness, and connection out of the picture. She thought, of course, that it was not right. She said that love, passion, creativity, playfulness, and connection were not left out, but dependent on her feeling attractive, which had to do with what Mark said and did.

Then I asked if she thought that a more loving connection could happen between people who were equal or people who were not equal. She thought it would be more likely between equals. If what Mark said and did determined how she felt, I wondered whether they could be on equal ground. She thought not, and found it disturbing that it was set up that way for her. I wondered, given the films, books, and ads that she mentioned, how many women could really not be affected by that kind of objectification. The answer 'not many' made sense to Victoria.

I asked Mark what it was like to listen to Victoria's conversation with me. He found it disturbing. He had always thought that Victoria was beautiful and did not know that she had such questions about it. This whole thing felt overwhelming.

This is a clear example of how we work to deconstruct dominant discourses. Jill's many questions opened space for Victoria to notice some of the ways that dominant stories about what constitutes beauty had seduced her and shaped her perceptions and beliefs. The power inequality between men and women around these discourses was also unmasked. Jill soon asked many similar questions to unpack the ways that Mark had been enrolled in patriarchal practices of power without realizing it.

In response to my questions about what he had learned while growing up as a boy and man about his role in a sexual relationship, Mark talked about the idea of conquest. Not having a sexual relationship with his wife for months had been humiliating to him as a man. I told him that I understood that it was common usage to say 'my wife', but said that to me it made Victoria sound more like a possession than a person. He could understand why it felt that way to me. I wondered whether the idea of a partner as a possession fit with conquest. He could see that it did, but hastened to add that of course he knew Victoria was a person. I agreed with him and wondered whether when it came to sex, the ideas of women as possessions and conquests that still circulate in the world had steered him away from his knowledge that Victoria was a person. He did not know.

We then began talking about what effects the idea that sex is conquest might have on him and on his relationship with Victoria. Mark thought the idea could put a lot of pressure on him to make sex happen. It could influence him to focus on quantity instead of quality. It could keep him from noticing his partner and what the experience was like for her. In some ways it would not matter what she did, as long as she was subservient. I wondered what he thought it would be like to be a woman in this kind of relationship. 'Like a prisoner', he said. 'Maybe if she were into S&M it would be great, but ...'

I talked about some of the ways everyday American culture gives men invitations to get caught up in this kind of thinking. Mark agreed that, without realizing it, he could have taken on some aspects of these ideas. He thought that this probably explained why he did not talk more before and during sex.

As she listened to my conversation with Mark, Victoria was able to look beyond the sadness and anger. She said that even though scrutinizing herself for attractiveness often got in the way, she and Mark had at times experienced profound connection and mutuality in sex. She described a particular experience, and on hearing her description Mark agreed it had been wonderful. They both remembered the communication and sense of partnership that were there. They agreed that their memories of this experience were a much better image of an intimate, sexual experience than any glamorized movie scene ever could be. I wondered how Victoria and Mark could keep the glamorized movie scenes out of their sex life. They thought that by paying attention to each other and communicating, they could be in charge of their sex life as partners. They agreed that they wanted to be in charge, instead of having unreal images and unjust ideas rule the sexual aspects of their relationship.

I saw Mark and Victoria three more times. They took the conversation about their sexual relationship very much to heart and felt a tremendous freedom to talk together about their feelings for each other and to try out new things in their ongoing sexual relationship. In the 12th and 13th meetings, they reflected on their unfolding sexual relationship. They told me how they had read poetry to each other in bed. Victoria was absolutely delighted with Mark's willingness to try new things. Mark was learning about himself and Victoria through these experiences. Victoria discovered that once she stopped worrying about how she looked and started noticing Mark, she became a very sexy woman! They both realized that fear had kept them comparing their relationship to an unreal standard. Now that the fear was gone, they both could see different possibilities for their sexual relationship. Victoria discovered that with the fear out of the way, it was easy to accept affection and be open. She wondered if Mark had actually offered more all along than she had known. Mark did not know. He said that although things were quite wonderful, he was struggling to have a voice without being authoritarian. We talked about the moments that he felt most able to do that, and resurrected some of the ideas from the last meeting that helped make that possible.

In the 12th meeting Victoria and Mark made a commitment to step out of what they were now seeing as the self-imposed limitations of their sexual relationship. Outside those bounds, they found laughter, safety, and good feelings, which they reported on at length in the 13th meeting. They agreed to talk with each other about the things they would be comfortable doing as well as those they would not be comfortable doing. They said they would find ways to 'try on' each other's desires.

Non-problematic narratives were clearly flowing again. Jill continued to ask questions to thicken the new stories as they emerged and did not have to be as active in structuring the interview. She could sit back and enjoy being part of this joyous conversation.

The 14th and last meeting was a time of looking back over what the couple had learned and accomplished. What stood out for Mark was that he did not have to be a leader, and not having to lead meant he could participate more. He thought he finally understood what Victoria meant by 'sharing dreams'. It did not have to do with creating grand plans. It had to do with being open about what was in his heart and mind. Victoria said that the biggest change for her had to do with realizing that she did not need someone who would open doors for her. She and Mark could go through them together.

Reflections on the work

In reviewing my notes, I am again grateful to Victoria and Mark for opening their lives to me and, through this writing, to all of us. The work with them did raise a number of dilemmas for me, some unique to their relationship and some common to work with many heterosexual couples. Because we shared both gender and social class, I was likely to understand and privilege Victoria's stories and understandings more than Mark's. Since I am a part of the dominant culture, there are many potentially limiting discourses that might have escaped my awareness. Reviewing my notes also reminded me of the power I wield in my role of questioner. Although questions are a tremendously valuable tool for collaboration, they still give the questioner power to propose conversational domains. With Mark and Victoria, I asked about the dilemmas of social class difference quite a bit before I asked about gender. I did not plan that sequence, but I am aware that I could have picked up on other strands of conversation that would have led us into considerations of gender sooner or of something else entirely. I was aware that I could have fallen into judgments of either Victoria for engaging in sexual relationships with people other than Mark or of Mark for being caught up in dominant ideas concerning men's sexuality as conquest. We think that either of these sets of judgements would have limited the usefulness of the therapy.

We hope that we have told the story of my work with Mark and Victoria with enough of the right kind of detail to give readers a feel for how we think and act in negotiating this terrain.

Note

1. We are not referring only to the full-blown diagnostic entity.

3

Gender stories[1]

This chapter was originally offered at a gender in therapy conference in the early 1990s. Looking back, this seems a long time ago and a great deal of thought and writing has occurred in relation to these issues since we wrote this paper. Nevertheless, we have included it here because it contains an exercise in relation to educating ourselves in recognising patriarchal culture and its effects, and we continue to hear from readers who tell us that they find this exercise very helpful.

Patriarchal gender stories interfere in men's and women's relationships. They support men (particularly white men) in a position of power and privilege in regard to women. The narrative therapist's task in regard to patriarchal stones is to highlight the gender roles that have developed from them, to ask questions to examine them and their implications more closely, and to create a context where people can begin to inhabit stories that offer more choice about their roles as men and women. The authors offer ideas about how to notice patriarchal stories and their influence, to recognize that other stories are possible, and to find collaborative, non-controlling ways of introducing conversation in this domain.

Years ago, one of the first times we went together to visit Gene's mother, something happened that neither of us would have predicted. We flew into Lexington, Kentucky, the airport nearest Pikeville, Gene's hometown, and rented a car for the two-and-a-half-hour drive from the bluegrass into the hills. At the end of our lushly scenic drive, Gene parked in a designated place on a sharp incline at the top of a steep hill and leaped out, anxious to see his mom. I (JF) was still sitting in the front seat gathering things together when the car started rolling backwards, down the hill. I was aware of the movement but it was as though I was paralyzed. Gene jumped for the door, managing to open it while the car continued its downhill progress. I sat frozen in the front seat, staring out at Gene. Finally, he was able to hurl himself into the car and hit the brakes. My hero!

What made each of us act as we did? What kept us from acting differently? There we were in a dangerous situation, our car hurtling down a treacherous hill. I (JF) could simply have slid across the seat and hit the brake. It would have been easy, and it is undoubtedly what I would have done if I had been alone. I (GC) could have assumed that Jill would have slid over and hit the brake or if she didn't, I could have alerted her to the situation. Something like, 'Hit the brakes!' probably would have done the trick. We believe that we acted as we did because we are part of a culture that has taught us all, men and women alike, to behave in particular ways based on our gender. Among other roles, men are taught to be in charge and women are taught to be in a supportive role – to be rescued, if you will. We tell this story to support our view that men are not the problem when it comes to men's and women's relationships. Neither are women. The culprit here is patriarchal culture (Eisler 1987; Hare-Mustin 1991).

The short-term effect on our lives of the event we have just recounted was that as we recovered from our intense embarrassment, we examined our relationship and compared the values that showed themselves in the incident with the values we aspire to live by. We think this has been helpful. The incident made us more aware of how cultural stories of male heroes rescuing females can dominate people's lives, perpetuating a society in which men control women and both women's and men's lives are limited. For us, it has become a priority to notice when we come under the influence of cultural stories that don't suit us and to struggle to author ones that suit us better.

The stories that circulate in our culture about women and men and what is possible between them are changing. Few of us have the same sort of relationships with our children, our friends, our partners, or ourselves that our parents did. The 'Leave it to Beaver/Father Knows Best' ideal that many of us grew up under is not the ideal for many people now. But the waning of the single-provider household and the rise of feminism have not meant the end of male domination, power, and privilege. Things are changing, but we all still swim in a sea of patriarchy.

Last summer some friends of ours became engaged. The four of us arranged to have dinner to celebrate. They came to our house first and from there we walked four or five blocks to a local restaurant. Carol and I (JF) walked side by side as did Gene and Brad. As we were walking Brad noticed a shorter route he could have taken and said, 'Oh, on the way to your house I should have turned back there'. Carol turned to me and in a hushed voice said, 'I knew that was the place to turn. But I was 'good', I didn't say anything.'

Carol and Brad had just become engaged, and this prompted me to think how incidents of this kind might become stories over the next 30 years of their marriage – stories of him being competent and her not, of his experience being privileged and hers devalued. I wondered what their children, if they have them, might learn about men's and women's roles from watching their parents. That a woman's job is to emotionally support men and make them feel good while she hides her own knowledge? That a man's role is to be the leader and the knower? And where did this idea that it was 'being good' to withhold knowledge come from?

We suggest that ideas like these come from the patriarchal system that we all live in.2 It was clear enough to Carol that this is the way things are that she leaned toward me and whispered conspiratorially, 'I knew that was the place to turn. But I was 'good', I didn't say anything.' And it was clear enough to me that this is the way things are that I, too, was 'good' and didn't say anything to Carol, although I was extremely uncomfortable.

Different roles for women and men

As we see it, there are two ways that patriarchal gender stories interfere in men's and women's relationships. One way is by promoting different sets of values and ways of being and the second way is by maintaining different levels of power and privilege.

If we look at values and ways of being, women, in general, are considered to value connection and relatedness and to be collaborative and intuitive. Men, in general, are thought of as competitive, rational, hierarchical, and valuing separation, autonomy, and strength. Women are said to express feelings and to describe particular experience and to be more interested in conversation as a process of connection and understanding. Men are said to give generalized, 'global' descriptions and to be more goal oriented in conversation (Belenky, Clinchy, Goldberger & Tarule 1986; Gilligan 1982; McLean 1992). Some people believe that these differences are absolute, that men and women have fundamentally different natures. We think of these differences as social constructions (Berger & Luckmann 1966; Gergen 1985); that is, we believe that they are prescribed and specified through generations of people in social interaction.

Mark, a college student who was seen by the training team at Evanston Family Therapy Center, gives us a glimpse of this process at work. Mark is suffering from a debilitating medical condition that not only keeps him in constant pain but severely restricts his activities. He has been talking about how it is now necessary for him to accept help from his friends in doing activities that previously would have been easy for him to do alone. The therapist, Ellen Taylor, asks him if it is hard to accept his friends' help. This is what Mark says:

MARK: Having my friends help me? That *is* hard. That's really hard for me. (Pause) *That also ties in to my upbringing.* I think I was always, well, my girlfriend says, hard core. I never laughed. I was really serious all the time. And I didn't need anything from anybody, you know. I was very independent – even when I was a teenager. I got to a point where I really didn't need anything, and I had a lot of people turn to *me.*

ELLEN: Where do you think that hard core, serious, independent way of being came from?

MARK: *It may have to do with being told what you're supposed to be as a man.* It's hard when you can no longer do a lot of those things. There was a lot of that at my high school. You had to be tough. And it's especially hard when I go home. I don't want to face people I knew, because I used to have ... I'm afraid I'll lose their respect because I no longer can … I can't defend myself anymore. Yeah, so, that's tough. I mean, right or wrong, it's hard.

This very astute young man is aware of the role the culture has played in defining masculinity, and he is painfully aware of how he doesn't fit the culture's definition.

We assert that few of us fit traditional gender stories throughout our lives, although most of us have distorted ourselves to try to fit those stories. We are 'good' and don't say what we know or we act in ways that don't fit who we are as people in hopes of 'fitting in'. A man who might have been a gentle and satisfied kindergarten teacher instead spends his life battling it out at the stock exchange. A woman who might have been director of a company instead (without recognition, status, or appropriate financial compensation) runs the company as the director's secretary.

Dominant gender stories, by their very dominance, restrain our imaginations and creativity. They specify normative roles for men and different normative roles for women. They construct anyone who lives outside their specifications as abnormal, perhaps as even sick or evil. They make it difficult for women and men to freely and fully collaborate in overcoming life's problems.

Different power for women and men

The second way that patriarchal stories interfere with men's and women's relationships is that they maintain gendered differences in power. Men (particularly white men) are in a position of power and privilege in regard to women in this culture. That is, men's experience and ideas are more valued in the culture than women's. Their domination, simply because of their gender, is built in (Goldner 1985; Goodrich 1991; Hare-Mustin 1987). The values of masculinity are built into the most powerful institutions in our society. To quote Christopher McLean (1992), who is researching the social construction of masculinity in Australia (but this certainly fits North America as well), 'The police, the military, political parties, the legal system and the media, all exhibit and enforce the characteristics of patriarchal masculinity. Big Business, universities, schools and sporting clubs all inculcate the masculine value of survival of the fittest, and select for success those who conform' (p. 8).

Marge, who I (GC) am seeing in therapy, speaks eloquently about this experience and its effects on her. She is struggling to overcome panic attacks and feelings of hopelessness. Just before the part of the conversation we will quote, she is telling about her work as a graphic artist and how even though one of her male clients treats her rudely and inconsiderately, she feels she must perform perfectly for him; she must please him at all costs. She then says that this habit of denying her own preferences in order to please powerful others is pervasive in her life. I ask her how she was recruited into this way of being. Here is her answer:

As I think about it, it's having lived in a culture where men were not accountable for anything they did. I grew up in a working-class family, and you were supposed to appease these men. And they did not have any obligation to understand. It was just accepted, they didn't understand anything. So you were just supposed to walk on eggshells and say the right thing. But you never had any idea what would happen.

It wasn't a sense of dealing with a rational person to whom you could say, 'Tuesday you said this and now you're saying this on Thursday'. It was like dealing with some kind of uncontrolled, unpredictable person. You know, who might be that way because he lost his temper, might be

> *that way because he was drunk, might be that way for any number of reasons, but this male person was in control of everything for no reason at all.*

I then mused aloud, saying that many people are now speaking out about this kind of subjugation. I asked her what she thought of her particular circumstances in the light of feminist critiques of our culture. Here's what she said:

> *Years ago I read* The Wounded Woman *(Leonard 1982). She talks about – to me it's a hard to grasp thing – about how women's very being was not acknowledged at all. It's different than being beaten or raped or whatever – having your very nature not acknowledged – and what happens to you because of that. I think it's true. I think that's part of what happened to me.*
>
> *It's very hard for me to perform in my profession unless I can get an 'A', unless I can get it perfect. It's like I'm looking at my clients and saying, 'Do they like me? Do they approve of me? Are they unhappy?' It's like I have to be directed outward all the time. It feels like that whole thing is about not having been acknowledged.*
>
> *And the thing about this dominant man is that you are always directed outward. You never know what anybody is going to say. You have to be directed outward just to be sure you don't get shot or something!*

If we think about the prevalence of stories like this in our culture, the idea that men and women can overcome gender-based differences by learning to accept, understand, and tolerate each other's values and ways of being is fraught with problems. We are not dealing with a simple matter of different-but-equal constructions of reality. Patriarchy values men's rights over women's rights. The dominant stories in our culture presuppose men's privilege and depict women as existing to support that privilege.

Let's take, for example, a heterosexual couple who often find themselves at odds because she approaches their conversations as a time for sharing feelings in a mutually supportive way and he approaches them as a time for solving problems. Cultural stories have taught both of them not only that his role is to do something about problems, but that problem solving is more important than is support or sharing. Each partner has been indoctrinated to believe that nurturing, supporting, and giving consolation are of secondary importance in this patriarchal culture where stories of action, accomplishment, and control reign supreme. Sharing feelings, nurturing, and giving consolation are part of being 'the woman behind the man'.

While the man in our example enjoys and benefits from the woman's fulfilment of her specified role, how can he really understand and value her way of being as a different-but-equal option? As long as dominant societal stories construct problem solving as more important than support and sharing, the man will have his way in their conversations – even though neither partner finds this truly satisfying.

As we have just implied, patriarchy has damaging effects on men as well as women. In specifying men's personhood patriarchy creates standards that may be difficult to live up to and it certainly limits men's choices. In heterosexual relationships it prevents them from having the experience of shared partnership with equals and the consequent possibility of enhanced intimacy (LaFollette 1992).

It is clear then that both women and men suffer under patriarchy. Unfortunately, patriarchy is a self-perpetuating system that will play no part in changing itself. Therefore, women and men together must take responsibility for standing up to patriarchy if we are ever to have a more just society. However, given our culture, where men have long been in a privileged position, where it is often unsafe for women to speak out about their experience, where separating themselves from oppressive lifestyles will often lead to physical as well as financial jeopardy, where significantly less risk is involved for men, and where women have long been leaders in speaking out against patriarchy, we believe that it is appropriate for men to take more of the responsibility for authoring new stories.

Our bias toward men taking more responsibility is reflected in our work. For example, since their marriage Tina and Jim had already moved twice to pursue job opportunities for Jim. Just as Tina finally began to feel settled in Chicago, Jim announced that he had earned a promotion that would take them to Dallas. They came to therapy because, upon hearing this news, waves of sadness and despondency came over Tina. She withdrew from the relationship and many of her newly established activities. She spent more and more time alone, doing less and less. Jim was concerned about Tina. He wondered if she would be able to take on the important jobs of organizing the move and orchestrating social activities with his new boss and colleagues.

We chose to start therapy with this couple by asking a series of questions about the beliefs and socialization processes that made Jim's job seem so important to him. We then asked questions that invited him to step into Tina's experience – to feel what it was like to be constantly moving from town to town in service to her husband's career. We could have started by asking how Tina could have a greater voice in the relationship, but since one of the culturally prescribed roles for women is 'caretaker of relationships', asking Tina to be more active in therapy would have preserved the status quo even as we sought to change it. As Jim began to understand how his behavior was influencing Tina, Tina did in fact speak out more for what was important to her.

The therapist's role in working with gender stories

In therapy guided by the narrative metaphor (Freedman & Combs 1994, 1996; White 1991; White & Epston 1990), we ask people to reflect on the stories that shape their lives. Therapy becomes a forum in which they can decide whether these stories really suit them as people. If they decide that the cultural stories do not fit for them, they are then free to engage with us in re-authoring their lives and relationships. The therapist's role in this process is to highlight limiting life narratives and the gender roles that have developed from them, to ask questions to examine those narratives and their implications more closely, and to create a context where people can begin to inhabit stories that offer more choice about their roles as men and women. We can summarize the process as one of deconstructing3 patriarchal stories and bringing forth new stories that offer expanded role choice.

Much has been written on the process of deconstructing limiting stories and bringing forth previously marginalized stories (Tomm 1989; White 1991; Zimmerman & Dickerson 1994). The challenge in using this process to promote non-patriarchal gender roles is to notice patriarchal stories and their influence, to recognize that other stories are possible, and to find collaborative, non-controlling ways of introducing conversation in this domain. Because we are all participants in the patriarchal culture, we will be blind to many of these possibilities.

For example, Fred, the father in one family in our live supervision program, sometimes yelled harshly at his children for little apparent reason. In therapy sessions, these outbursts would end with the children crying and the adults sitting in silence. After each of these incidents, the therapist proceeded as though nothing had happened. As the team reflected on a particular session, the possibility was broached that limiting gender stories might be coaching Fred's outbursts, the children's crying, and the silence of the other adults. The therapist responded that she thought these ways of being were okay with the family. She said that it sounded as if the team were trying to impose 'politically correct' feminist values on her and on the family. However, the next time these behaviors occurred, she began to ask questions about them. The family members, including Fred, each noted their unhappiness with the yelling and the tense silence that always followed it. Then the parents, responding to further questions, went on to describe how their gender socialization had contributed to these ways of being. After the session, the therapist said, 'I didn't recognize what was happening as a problem. Maybe I just wanted Fred to like me.' She then went on to reflect on how certain gender stories had influenced her to want Fred to like her and had kept her from seeing this as a problem.

Because we are participants in a patriarchal culture, gender stories and their effects offer a challenge for all of us. We are often blind to them, and the people we work with don't often name them as problems, even when they experience their effects as problematic. Even when we do recognize them, our own socialization may inhibit us from talking about them.

It is important that therapists begin to recognize gender stories as they are being lived out and described and that they have ways of initiating conversations about them. In pursuit of these goals, we offer three practices that are central to our work in re-authoring gender stories with people:

1. Educating ourselves to recognize patriarchal culture and its effects.
2. Listening for discrepancies that might open onto non-patriarchal gender stories.
3. Asking questions that might bring forth non-patriarchal gender stories.

Educating ourselves to recognize patriarchal culture and its effects

Rachel Hare-Mustin (1994) likens the therapy room to a room with mirrored walls, reflecting back only what is said inside it. 'If the therapist and family are unaware of marginalized discourses, such as those associated with members of subordinate gender, race, and class groups', she notes, 'those discourses remain outside the mirrored room' (p. 22).

In our quest to bring more discourses into the therapy room, we have found it helpful to read feminist literature, to participate in discussions about patriarchal culture, and to reflect on the effects of patriarchal culture in people's life stories, including our own. We offer the following set of questions as an example of how we invite people who attend our workshops into this sort of discussion and reflection. Although one person can consider the questions on his or her own, we believe they work best in a discussion group with each person in the group getting a chance to respond to a question before the group moves on to the next question. This facilitates an interweaving of people's individual stories,4 giving a richer sampling of the cultural gender discourse each story is part of. We ask participants to wait until the end to respond to each other's stories. We want people to have an experience of their stories unfolding. This seems more likely to happen if participants go through the entire structured experience before stepping out of it to reflect on it.

1. You have probably reflected at times on how relationships in your local culture (if not at home then at school, the neighborhood, religious institutions, the media, etc.) modeled gender roles for you. What *specific incident* that is illustrative of this process stands out for you?

2. What was the meaning of this incident (and others like it) to you? What generalizations did such incidents invite you to make? Did it influence you to form any beliefs about how women should be in relation to men or to each other? How men should be in relation to women or to other men? Or about power and privilege?

3. How have the ways of being that were modeled for you by incidents like the one you related influenced your relationships with men (both personally and

as a therapist)? How have they influenced your relationships with women (both personally and as a therapist)? What has been positive about this and what has been negative about this?

4. What is an example of a time you were able to act outside of the limits prescribed for you by the incident you have been talking about? Tell the story of a particular incident.

5. How were you able to take the stand that you did against the old ways of being? What does it mean that you were able to act as you did in this new incident? What characteristics does it show that you have? (What name would you give to this newer way of being?)

6. What did you learn in the process that has been helpful to you personally? What did you learn that is helpful in working with people in therapy?

7. What possibilities will it open for your future if this way of being becomes more and more available to you? What do you see as the next step in this progression?

8. How would relationships between men and women that you work with in therapy be different if this way of being was part of the dominant societal stories about gender?

After a group has finished the last question we offer people an opportunity to respond to anything they have heard from each other. A discussion may then follow about thoughts and ideas people had in going through the process.

We have outlined this exercise as an example of one way that therapists can develop awareness both of gender stories that have limited them in the past and of how they have transcended the limits of those stories. The more stories of transcendence we can bring into the mirrored room of therapy, the less we will be limited by patriarchal discourse.

Listening for discrepancies that might open onto non-patriarchal gender stories

Once a therapist is attuned to the influence of patriarchal gender narratives, it is important to be able to introduce conversations that open space for marginalized exceptions to those stories. As people speak in ways that seem prescribed by the patriarchal culture,[5] we listen for discrepancies in the story and in the ways of being that it prescribes. Statements such as, 'They know I'd wallop them if you weren't here', and 'She knows I value how she takes care of everything at home but my job is more important because the money I make makes everything else possible' are examples of statements containing the kind of discrepancies we're talking about. Although they represent the dominant gender discourses, they indicate at least an awareness of other possibilities. We can bring the other possibilities into the conversation by asking about them.

Consider this conversation:

MAUREEN: I think we need a budget we both agree on so that we only spend what we can afford.

DAN: (To the therapist) She wouldn't dare say that if you weren't here.

THERAPIST: What would happen if she said that when the two of you were alone?

DAN: I'd tell her no and if she kept it up I'd walk out.

THERAPIST: What keeps you from doing that here?

DAN: You know, I'm trying to be reasonable.

THERAPIST: Does that mean if she said that at home and you told her no and then walked out, you would be being unreasonable?

DAN: Well, I earn much more than she does, so what right does she have telling me what to do with my money?

THERAPIST: Let's slow this down a little bit. Why do you think it would be unreasonable for you to say no when Maureen brings up the budget?

DAN: Because if we are going to have a good relationship we need to be able to discuss things.

THERAPIST: Okay, so you think it would be best if the two of you could have a reasonable discussion about your budget?

DAN: Yeah, I guess so.

THERAPIST: So, I'm confused. What keeps you from wanting to have that discussion outside of my presence?

DAN: I don't know. I'm doing all this work and I'm the one who makes most of the money that we live on, so I should be in charge.

We now have statements indicative of two different stories. We can begin to deconstruct the dominant story based on patriarchal values by asking Dan questions such as the following: Where did you learn that money should determine who is in charge? What gives paid work more value then unpaid work? Who supports those views and who does not? What effect has it had on your relationship to think that you should be in charge?

We can help co-author an alternative story by focusing on Dan's statement that it would be best if they could have a reasonable discussion about their budget. We might ask Maureen questions like: Are you surprised to hear Dan say that he thinks it would be best if the two of you discussed your budget reasonably? What values does that let you know he has? If you look into your past, what times stand out for you that demonstrate that he has these values? What kind of hope does that give you for the relationship? Does that hope encourage you to do anything that you have not done before or haven't done lately? Such questions invite both Maureen and Dan into an experiential exploration of a less patriarchal story for their future. In order to ask these questions, the therapist had to notice the useful discrepancy in Dan's statement, 'She wouldn't dare say that if you weren't here'.

Asking questions that might bring forth non-patriarchal gender stories

In the above example, discrepancies that could be openings for marginalized gender stories occurred spontaneously in conversation. When such openings don't seem to appear we can often bring them to light by asking questions. Rick Maisel (1994) has suggested two kinds of inquiry that seem relevant in this regard. One is to ask people about their intentions and then attend to contradictions between their intentions and the actual effects of their behavior. In this sort of inquiry, a father who often doesn't show up for activities he has planned with his children might be asked about the intentions that guided his decision to do something else. If he says that he was responding to the needs of important clients so that he wouldn't lose their business, and that his intention in doing that was to provide security for his family, the therapist could then inquire about the effects of his repeated 'no-shows' on his children's sense of security.

The second kind of inquiry that Maisel suggests is to attend to the contradiction between a belief and the effects of that belief on a particular relationship. For example, if a man believes that it is wrong to burden other people with his worries, a therapist could ask questions that invited him to examine the effects of his silence in several areas of his marital relationship. How does it affect problem-solving discussions? How does it affect his ability to share hopes and enthusiasms? Does it have positive or negative effects on the couple's sexual relationship? Such inquiry would almost certainly open space for authoring stories that could support a new belief about what to do with worries. We have found both of these lines of inquiry useful in bringing forth discrepancies that can then open onto new gender stories.

We would like to suggest a third kind of questioning – contrasting one context with another. If we can find a context where a person is less influenced by patriarchal dictates, we might be able to help examine the relationship in the light of that context.

For example, I (JF) recently saw a couple who were discouraged and disconcerted by the anger and misunderstanding that was coming between them. Anne described her life as divided between her work as a professor, which included a research project and a book in progress, and primary responsibility both for running the household and for parenting the couple's two children. Jeffrey was also a professor and had comparable professional responsibilities. He said that he was quite willing, in fact wanted, to help around the house. The problem, as Anne described it, was that being in charge of the house and the children made her feel frazzled and impatient. This contributed to anger and misunderstandings. They knew that the obvious solution was to give Jeffrey more responsibilities. However, they believed that this was not possible because Anne saw things that Jeffrey did not. They both believed that she was intrinsically an organized person and that he was not. Jeffrey was glad to step in when she asked, but they both believed that if he took charge of any of the overseeing, important things would be overlooked.

It was at this point that I decided to ask about another context. Since I knew that both Jeffrey and Anne were self-directed in their work, I decided to ask questions about their offices. Jeffrey's office, it turned out, was immaculate – completely organized in a system he developed that worked smoothly. Anne's office, on the other hand, looked like a disaster area. She described stacks of papers, piles of books, and no real system of organization. In the work context, Jeffrey always met deadlines. Anne did not. He seemed to know what needed doing when. She often felt behind.

After hearing these descriptions I asked if they could understand how I now had a different picture of both of them. I asked if they could see how this new picture put the idea of Anne being the intrinsically organized one, the one who was a perfect overseer, into a different light. They could. I then wondered with them what had contributed to their household roles as they had developed. They began to see how gender socialization had played a big part in this. We were then in a position to examine the stories that supported their gender socialization and to discuss the effects of those stories on their relationship. This let them begin to live out stories in which they each experienced more choice about how to share their roles as homemakers and parents.

The contrast between qualities people show in different contexts is not always this extreme. However, we have found that our believing that these qualities are not intrinsic but are socially constructed helps us find differences in different contexts. This skill, like the others we have mentioned, flows from therapists' efforts not to allow themselves to be blinded by patriarchy.

In summary, we believe that the dominant stories about how men and women should be can change. We believe it because we have seen changes of this kind taking place – not in the dominant culture but in the local cultures of families with whom we have worked. In therapy, as people realize that taken-for-granted gender stories are not essential truths, but social constructions that can be changed, they are standing up to those stories. They then begin to discover events and ideas at variance with the previously unquestioned stories, thus glimpsing new possibilities. As they move toward the new possibilities, they rediscover moments in their lives and relationships that suit them. As they use these moments to construct and inhabit stories that take back their lives from the constricting influence of patriarchal culture, they help bring forth a different kind of culture with more room for all of us.

We believe that it is important to circulate the unique stories that people choose to live out as widely as possible. Only as stories that support alternative ways of being become more widely available will patriarchal stories cease to dominate us.

Notes

1. An earlier draft of this article was presented as a Plenary Address at the 'Bridging the Gender Gap' conference sponsored by the Chicago Center For Family Health on February 18 & 19, 1994. This paper was first published in Journal of Systemic Therapies, Vol. 15, No. 1, Spring 1996.
2. When we use the word patriarchy, which Carol Gilligan (statement made at the *Learning From Women* conference, Boston, 1993) has noted is another word for civilization, we are referring to a system of values, beliefs, and practices that maintain certain small numbers of people in positions of power over large numbers of other people, according to distinctions such as race, class, sexual orientation, and gender.
3. By *deconstructing* we mean a process of 'unpacking' stories and their implications. This involves looking at how those stories were constructed and passed on in people's local cultures (which requires that people see their stories as constructions rather than received truths). It also involves examining the effects of the stories on people's lives and relationships.
4. The idea of interweaving individual stories was sparked by JF's attendance at a Public Conversations Project workshop where Sallyann Roth and Dick Chasin facilitated such an experience.
5. The more we educate ourselves about patriarchal culture and its effects, the more we see the relevance of gender stories in whatever problems bring people to therapy.

4

Minimizing Hierarchy in Therapeutic Relationships

A reflecting team approach[1]

by

S. Michele Cohen, Gene Combs, Bill DeLaurenti, Pat DeLaurenti, Jill Freedman, David Larimer, Dina Shulman

This chapter was created through a collaborative process which we still treasure. A heterosexual couple who were coming for therapy (Bill DeLaurenti and Pat DeLaurenti), a number of therapists (Michele Cohen, David Larimer and Dina Shulman), and ourselves (who were acting as supervisors) all came together to collaborate on a conference presentation and then this article. The process was extremely rigorous. More importantly, it was experientially congruent with the subject of the paper – the value of minimizing hierarchy in therapeutic relationships. More time was probably spent creating this article than any other we have worked on. The process of collaboration was unique, at least in our experience. We learned so much from it and the process was highly valued by everyone involved. It's a great pleasure to be able to include this paper here.

What we report here is a work in progress – our team's description of practices that served to minimize hierarchies in working together over the course of a particular therapy and of the effects these practices have had on us both personally and professionally. In what follows, we will introduce ourselves and describe our approach, share some personal reflections about our experience, and then offer some questions that we have found useful and important. Our intention (see Combs & Freedman 1994) is to invite readers to reflect upon the impact of how hierarchy may be structured in their own therapeutic work and to suggest some ways – and reasons – we have found for socially constructing therapeutic relationships that minimize hierarchy. When the seven of us began working together, we didn't know that our labor would be so long, so challenging, or so rewarding.

The Team

Our team came together in the course of a live supervision program in narrative therapy (Freedman & Combs 1996; Monk, Winslade, Crocket & Epston 1997; White 1991, 1995a; White & Epston 1990; Zimmerman & Dickerson 1996) using a reflecting team format (Andersen 1987, 1991; Friedman 1995; White 1995b). Members included Pat and Bill DeLaurenti, a couple who came to consult about problems in their relationship; Michele Cohen, Dina Shulman, and David Larimer, who had signed on for supervision of their work; and Jill Freedman and Gene Combs, who had offered the supervision. Michele and Dina each served as therapists at different points in the process and reflecting team members at other times. David was a member of the reflecting team throughout. Gene and Jill at different times were either members of the reflecting team or supervisors.

When this team first met, Jill and Gene had been working for several years to set up structures and practices that might minimize hierarchy in their narrative therapy supervision program. Michele, Dina, and David were a group of supervisees who fully embraced the collaborative and egalitarian ways of working proposed. Pat and Bill learned of our program through David, who was seeing Pat individually. Both members of the couple had some initial reservations, but they agreed to come for three sessions.[2] After the agreed-upon sessions, Pat and Bill decided to continue. They found that participating in a process where their ideas and opinions were valued and where they had the opportunity to listen in on the thoughts of the therapists made the experience of therapy less blaming and demeaning than they had feared it might be. The entire team met every other week for a total of eleven sessions.[3]

We have been fortunate in this project to have been able to take the team process a bit further than any of us had before by continuing to meet as a team outside of the therapy. When the formal supervision program ended, we were all so pleased by the experience that we decided to offer a workshop together on minimizing hierarchy. Our proposal was accepted for the Narrative Ideas and Therapeutic Practice conference in Vancouver in 1997. Planning for that presentation gave us more experience in working together as a collaborative group, and the presentation in March was so well received that we decided to continue working together to write this paper.

The entire group met three times over a four-month period to discuss the form and content of this paper. We agreed that Pat, Bill, Michele, Dina, and David would each write several pages that gave a snapshot of what they found important and memorable about the work we did together. Jill and Gene would then put those pieces together with some thoughts of their own, and the whole paper would be circulated to all group members for comment and revision.

Jill and Gene's introduction

As you will see throughout this chapter, we have minimized hierarchy in a number of ways, but we have not eliminated it altogether. As the people who set up this situation in the beginning, the two of us continue to have a somewhat bigger voice and to bear somewhat more of the responsibility for what happens. If you, as a reader of this paper, have ideas about how we might make our work more collaborative and egalitarian, we would love to hear from you. Before we talk about *why* we are interested in minimizing hierarchy, we would like to describe the structure our team followed as we worked together and some of the practices we used within that structure.

The Structure

We scheduled two hours for each meeting, and we divided that time into the following segments (see 'Structure of our team process'):

A *presession meeting* between therapist and supervisor, with the couple and the team listening in from behind the mirror. The therapist typically used this time with the supervisor to develop the story of her own struggles and growth as a therapist. As a part of this conversation, she would identify things that she would like the team to reflect on as they observed her work on that particular evening. This presession meeting lasted about twenty minutes.

A *therapy session,* lasting about an hour, in which the therapist interviewed the couple. The team, including the supervisor, was behind the mirror.

About forty minutes into the therapy session, there was a break for a *reflecting team* (Freedman & Combs 1996; White 1995b). In the reflecting team format, first developed by Tom Andersen (1987, 1991), the team observing the therapy session switches places with the therapist and family (or client) and has a conversation that the therapist and family observe. Then, after switching places again, the family comments on the team's reflections. At this point in our structure, the couple and therapist joined the supervisor behind the mirror while the rest of the team members went in front of the mirror and reflected on what they noticed and what they were curious about in the therapy. Reflections usually focused on some alternative story that the couple was developing.

After the reflecting team had met for about ten minutes, the therapist and the couple resumed their places in front of the mirror for ten minutes or so to talk about what stood out for them from the reflecting team's comments.

Then there was a *post-therapy meeting* for about twenty minutes, which took different forms at different times at the discretion of the therapist. Sometimes the reflecting team would reflect on the therapist's work and the therapist would reflect on the team's reflections. At other times the supervisor would interview the therapist to develop her story of herself as a therapist. The couple and other team members observed from behind the mirror.

Each two-hour session ended with twenty minutes or so of *post-therapy deconstruction* (Madigan 1993; White 1995b), where everyone involved sat together in the same room. Anyone could ask questions of the therapist or reflecting team members about the thoughts and intentions that shaped what they did and didn't do in the session.

We believe that several things about this structure serve to minimize hierarchy. The presession conversation demystifies and de-deifies therapists. As people who have come for help listen in on the therapist and supervisor, they can experience the therapist as a growing, developing practitioner who, like them, is striving to bring forth preferred ways of being in the world. The reflecting team assures that team members do their thinking, planning, and discussing out loud, in front of the people who have come for help, again demystifying the therapists' ideas. The post-therapy deconstruction gives space for everyone to evaluate each session, question any other member of the team about his or her motives and intentions, and examine the effects of what was or wasn't done.

Structure of our team process

1. *Presession Meeting* (20 minutes)
   Therapist and supervisor talk in front of mirror, family and reflecting team listen behind mirror.
2. *First Part of Therapy Session* (about 40 minutes)
   Team and supervisor listen behind mirror while therapist and family talk in front.
3. *Reflecting Team* (about 10 minutes)
   Therapist, family, and supervisor listen behind mirror while team talks in front.
4. *Second Part of Therapy Session* (about 10 minutes)
   Team and supervisor listen behind mirror while therapist and family reflect on team's reflections in front.

5. *Post-Therapy Meeting* (about 20 minutes)
   Either:
   Reflecting team reflects on therapist's work, then therapist and supervisor reflect on their reflections.
   Or:
   Supervisor interviews therapist to bring forth story of his or her development as a therapist.
6. *Post-Therapy Deconstruction* (about 20 minutes)
   Everyone asks therapist and reflecting team members questions to deconstruct their intentions and motivations in the session. (Everyone is in front of mirror.)

Note: All times in this table are approximate. In practice, the times varied according to the desires of the participants.

The practices

Perhaps the most important contribution therapists can make to minimizing hierarchies is an intangible one that has to with taking on particular presuppositions, both about the people we work with and about the therapist's role. We believe that the people we work with are knowledgeable about what is helpful and meaningful in their struggles. We assume that our role calls for some expertise in asking questions, but it does not imply that we are experts on other people's problems or on how they should think, act, or feel. Our way of being with people stems from and conveys these presuppositions. We hope that our manner, tone of voice, posture, and the like invite people to enter into collaborative therapeutic relationships with us.

Additionally, there are a number of things that we do intentionally to minimize hierarchies:

- *Not talking about people outside of their presence,* a practice built into the structure we have just described, is exceedingly helpful in maintaining the kind of respect that makes collaborative partnerships work. We find that over time this practice shapes not only what therapists do, but what they think.

- *Reflecting teams,* in which therapists respond to new developments in people's lives while those people observe, have transformed the way many therapeutic teams work. It was an important part of how our team worked in this project.

- *Asking questions* rather than making statements sets the whole tone of therapy and contributes to a context in which the voices of the people who have come to consult with us are honored. As Karl Tomm (1988) points out, asking questions defines the domain of 'appropriate' answers, but the answerer draws on his or her own ideas, knowledge, and values in constructing answers. Asking questions from a position of genuine 'curiosity' (Cecchin 1987) or 'not-knowing' (Anderson 1990; Anderson & Goolishian 1992) is essential if questions are to actually function to help minimize hierarchies.

- *Striving to not make assumptions* also helps minimize hierarchy. We try to notice things we are taking for granted, and to question them, so that we don't unwittingly construct the therapy on our own taken-for-granted worldview. We believe that this minimizes the tendency for us to impose our values and beliefs on people. We know that this simple-sounding practice is humanly impossible to achieve fully, but we believe that striving for it is worthwhile.

  One way of inviting others to question our assumptions is through what Michael White (1991) has called *transparency.* In practicing transparency we let people in on the experiences that shape our thoughts and intentions rather than presenting them as expert knowledge. A benefit of working with a team is that team members can ask each other *situating questions.* These questions invite team members to identify and describe the experiences, intentions, and motivations that shape their contributions to the therapy, thus making them more transparent. We find that questioning each other and being questioned develops habits of self-reflection that carry over into those more typical contexts in which we work alone. It helps us to be more explicit, even when we aren't working with a team, about where our ideas come from, what our intentions are, and what our values and biases are.

- *Including the people who consult us in presession and postsession meetings* invites them to join the team in planning, deconstructing, and evaluating the therapy. They see therapists struggling with their own stories in a process similar to therapy. This invites them to perceive the therapists as people, rather than as experts. We have found it particularly useful to ask clients to evaluate therapy. Not only do we get invaluable guidance and direction from these evaluations, we can also look back at our work through different eyes and see 'sparkling moments' we have not seen before.

Pat reflects

When I walked in for our first session I wasn't sure what was going to happen, so I felt very uncomfortable. As the sessions continued, I felt more at ease and looked forward to the next one. It was different for me than most of my sessions with doctors or therapists over the years. At most of my previous sessions I felt like I was a very small person and the doctors and therapists were giants. I felt they were better and smarter than me. You see, I have always put them up on pedestals.

What was different for me in this new setting was that at every session I learned that you are not just a client and a therapist, you are a team working together for the same end result. The other team members are not better than me, they are human like me – even though Bill and I were the clients and they were the therapists, and one might usually be seen as outranking the other. As the sessions went on I felt that the gap between everyone got smaller and smaller. That's when we became a team or a family working together. I feel because of this the end result was achieved sooner.

Being present during the pre- and postsessions and the reflecting team discussions made therapy more comfortable. During the presession you got to see what to expect during the session, about how it might be done differently to improve the quality of the session for both client and therapist. When it was time to switch for the reflecting team it was even better. You could see how everybody sees things differently. We got instant feedback and input about our session. We were also included, if we wanted to be, in the postsession. We all sat in a circle and discussed how the session went. As clients we were able to give our opinions about how the session went and to comment on anything the therapist did well or could improve on.

Was there anything I could suggest to improve this process? I'd have to say no, because I have never been in that kind of situation before. I was glad to be a part of this process. Everyone benefitted from it. We all learned from this. Gene and Jill were learning how to better shorten the bridge between supervisor and therapist. The therapists also learned how to shorten the bridge between themselves and their clients. All to improve the quality of the outcome.

I was excited when I was asked if I would like to be included in the presentation of this process, but I wasn't sure how I wanted to be a part of it. I attended the planning meetings and gave input and feedback. The only way I felt comfortable to participate in the Vancouver conference was to write this in the form of a letter, which has now become my contribution to this paper. I am glad to have this opportunity to help others see how important it is to shorten the bridge or, as they say, 'minimize the hierarchy'.

Bill reflects

I became a team player in a rather strange way. Pat's psychiatrist (a hierarchy person) told her that if she wanted to continue seeing her, Pat and I would have to go to counseling. I was planning on not doing this, but then her counselor (David, whom I had confidence in) suggested this group.

At first I was a little unsure of what was going to be done. After things got under way, I felt more comfortable. Even though you knew others were watching, you felt more relaxed than if you were just with one person. I really didn't know why this was at first, but as time went by, I realized that it was because we were becoming a team (also friends). We were all pretty much on the same platform.

Because of the presession, postsession, and reflecting team, there was a lot more input and feedback. Things seemed to move along smoothly, because of so many team players. Things were made clearer because we checked in with one another every so often. While watching the presession, you sometimes would learn what the student and supervisor thought of previous meetings and what they might want to try next. Every time the reflecting team talked, many more questions or comments were brought up. I believe because of the reflecting team, the conversation seemed more equal to us, the clients.

It felt good knowing that even while you were learning new and helpful things, you were also helping the students and the supervisors learn some new things. Even though supervisors have more knowledge of the process, you felt more like you had an equal voice. This was unlike some one-on-ones that I have experienced. It was also nice to hear how the team thought we were doing and where they saw us going. It was great to be able to get some suggestions on what we could try to possibly improve things rather than to be told what we have to do.

It seemed that after every meeting, on our way home, we would continue talking about what we had learned and what we could possibly do to improve our situation even more. I think this was because we felt more comfortable or positive with ourselves.

Dina reflects

The process of doing what we call therapy can be rewarding or frustrating, empowering or oppressing, energizing or isolating. What determines this difference in experience? I have struggled to decipher what exactly 'it' is – what influences people's experience of therapy. Not only what influences me, as a clinician, but what influences my clients. Is 'it' the same for every person? I continue to struggle. However, during this supervision program and my work with Pat, Bill, Michele, David, Gene, and Jill, I began to develop some ideas of what 'it' is for me.

The team and I had been working with Pat and Bill for about a month when – during my presession – Jill and I were discussing thoroughness in therapy. Jill wondered what might get in the way of my being thorough during the upcoming session. We found that excitement at times gets me to leap forward and move too fast, leaving the people I am working with confused and frustrated. We also discussed ways in the past that I might have stood up to the negative effects of excitement by checking in with my clients and clarifying with them what I was hearing. Michele, David, Gene, Pat, and Bill were witnesses to this discussion through a one-way mirror.

As foreseen, excitement showed up full force during the session. Pat and Bill were discussing the times when their communication together worked. I saw them making great strides and wanted them to realize the magnitude of what they were saying. At one point, I found myself sitting on the edge of my chair, leaning forward, asking question upon question to build on this new story I was hearing. I realized that I was not fully listening to their answers before asking another question. I somehow stopped myself and said, 'Am I jumping ahead? I'm getting excited ....' Another time during the session I found my mind racing forward once again. I could not seem to formulate any question that made sense, so I just said, 'Am I getting excited? Would you like me to rephrase the question?'

After each of these examples I was met with smiles (and maybe a little relief) from Pat and Bill. I heard some friendly laughter from the team through the mirror. Encouraged by those responses, I was able to slow down and start again unencumbered by overexcitement.

During my conversation with Jill in the post-therapy meeting, we reflected on this experience. The first thought that came to me was, 'What a luxury!' Knowing that Pat and Bill had heard the conversation about excitement in the presession, knowing that they knew about my goals for the therapy session, was really helpful. Having support for saying out loud, 'Oh, no, I think I'm getting excited' allowed me to be clear and unapologetic about what was happening and to involve Pat and Bill in the discussion about what to do instead of trying to do all this secretly in my head. I felt mildly embarrassed, but I did not feel incompetent.

The freedom to speak openly and honestly also seemed to help me focus. I was able to readjust and ask an appropriate question without losing contact by withdrawing into a private (and probably overly critical) conversation with myself. With everyone involved, I was filled and gratified with a sense of teamwork.

At first, the idea of having my clients witness discussions of my struggles and fears as a therapist was daunting. I wondered how these people would think that I could help them if they were to know my insecurities and struggles. I was anxious. I had to fight the grip of societal ideas about what a therapist should know and how a therapist should act.

It helped to remember times I have felt quite isolated, working alone in my office hour after hour. The idea of working with my clients as a team seemed like a natural antidote to isolation. As I confronted the anxiety and took some risks, I found myself working in a freeing, comfortable, and educational environment. I didn't just *think about* working as a team with the people who came to consult me, I actually did it. We all helped each other.

In the beginning of my work as a therapist I had felt that I had to play the expert therapist who knew all the answers to any problem. I had always felt uncomfortable in this role, but I thought that people would want that from me. From the moment I started learning about narrative therapy, I have tried to avoid the role of expert, but it was not until I experienced Pat and Bill observing my struggles as a therapist that I could know that I was really shedding this costume.

During the training program I was supported in working with a high degree of transparency, sharing my thoughts and struggles with my colleagues and clients. As this transparency grew, I was able to relax and do my work without worrying about acting like an 'appropriate therapist'. Pat and Bill told us that it made them feel better to know that their therapist was human and had problems of her own. They said that when they didn't have to relate to us as experts, when they could treat us as actual human beings who were learning from them as well as helping them, they felt more comfortable.

Most of the time, one does not have the luxury of working with a reflecting team and being supervised before and after a session. Since the training program ended, I have tried to incorporate these ideas when working on my own. I have continued to see Pat and Bill in counseling, and by constantly checking in with them, I feel that we have become a collaborative team. They let me know when I let excitement rush me. I consult with them to be sure we are still moving in the direction that they want. They seem to feel comfortable letting me know when something has been helpful and when something has not. I look forward to seeing Pat and Bill more than I used to look forward to sessions when I thought I was working alone. I find our sessions more productive. I know that when I see Pat and Bill we will struggle *together* to figure out how to make our therapy experience as helpful and comfortable as possible.

David reflects

To clearly illustrate how working with Pat, Bill, Dina, Michele, Jill, and Gene continues to shape me and my work with clients, it is important to provide some background information. For the past few years I had been working with Pat on an individual basis, occasionally seeing her with Bill. There were also occasions when I saw Pat and Bill along with their two children. As I had worked with Pat in that period, I believed that I had always treated her with respect and always thought we were working together in this process.

Approximately eight months prior to the time that Pat and Bill and I began working with the team, I had been hearing repeatedly from Pat that our work together was going in circles. At the time what I believed was that Pat wasn't listening to me or doing the things I thought she needed to do to move ahead. Consequently, I continued to hear Pat say during those eight months that we were going in circles.

Interestingly enough, about six months after we had completed our presentation in Vancouver, Pat made the statement that we were again going in circles. This time by the end of the session we were able to make some changes that appeared to have us moving in a different direction, not merely going in circles. Pat and I have since had several conversations about what was different this time from the first time.

We believe that as a result of working with the team I have been developing a much clearer understanding of how people can work collaboratively and of the power of genuine curiosity. This has had big effects on the way I listen to Pat. This time I wasn't trying to convince Pat to accept my version of what she wasn't doing or what she needed to do. Instead, I was influenced by a belief that it was important to listen with curiosity. As Pat talked about what she thought was inviting us to go around in circles and what she believed could help us get out of going around in circles, it appeared that we were developing more of a partnership. We were making therapy more useful and finding a direction that both she and I would prefer.

In our work with the team I have seen myself take some ideas of narrative therapy (such as collaboration, curiosity, and avoiding expert knowledge) and feel them come alive in my relationship with Pat and with other people.

There is a growing belief in collaboration that encourages Pat and me to have regular conversations about what is working, what we would prefer to work on, and how to go about doing that. This work continues to be transforming and challenging. It shapes the way I listen and what I listen to, adding complexity and subtlety to my understanding of the power of curiosity and of minimizing hierarchy in my relationships with others.

Michele reflects

As a narrative therapist, I am interested in collaborating with people to minimize the influence of problems in their lives. One of the things that attracted me to the narrative approach was that it would support me in working as a team member, sharing my impressions, ideas, and agendas, and asking people's guidance in correcting my errors and misbeliefs. I like relating to the people who consult with me as a person who is in it with them rather than as an expert who evaluates their situation from a professional distance and then tells them the correct way to act, think, and feel.

In the session that I want to focus on, I experienced Pat as confronting Bill about a problem that plagued their relationship. She stated that she felt very upset that Bill constantly walked in front of her, not side-by-side. She compared this to the way a master and servant would walk. She said that one effect of this problem was to make her feel 'not quite equal, like a little kid' and as if Bill 'just doesn't care'. She believed that this pattern had been going on for a long time. Pat seemed to be saying that she felt like she was one-down in a hierarchical relationship, and that this feeling brought on the further feeling that Bill didn't care for her. Even though Bill refuted the claim, stating that he was 'just a fast walker,' it seemed to me that Pat was glimpsing a preferred direction for her life with Bill. I was curious to hear more about this new direction and the possibilities Pat thought it might offer.

The situation that Pat described with Bill is just the sort of situation that our team is working to avoid in therapeutic relationships. We want the people who consult us to feel that they are our equals and that we care about them and their situations. At the time of this session, I was just beginning to notice and try to deconstruct the societal influences that might lead me to feel or act expert or 'one-up' with people who were consulting me. Asking questions to explore what supported hierarchy and what its effects were in Pat and Bill's relationship gave me an opportunity to grapple with its supports and effects in my own life as a therapist.

In the first reflecting team (we had two in this particular therapy session) Jill wondered if Pat knew that other women shared her feeling of being like a servant or a little kid rather than like an equal partner in their marriages. This question invited me to think about the societal supports of hierarchy, and to use that mind-set in the rest of the session. Since that session, a concern with societal influences has become a more direct part of my work. I am more and more able to ask questions that help me break the grip of societal assumptions on my eyes and ears and in turn on the eyes and ears of those I work with.

After the first reflecting team, Pat was able to share that she was not aware of the notion that other women shared this experience. She was intrigued to hear that she was not alone. I wondered out loud about what possibilities this knowledge opened up for her. She wondered how other women handled it. In response to further questions from me, Pat talked about having a dream, 'just a dream', that one day she would take the lead when she and Bill were shopping. She would know what she wanted to do, to see, and to buy. Bill would follow *her* for a change.

It was encouraging for me to hear these ideas from Pat. It raised interesting new questions in my mind. How might this dream help her to challenge hierarchy if it showed up in other contexts? Would this experience allow her to feel more equal in our work? Would she be able to let me know if I was 'taking the lead' too much?

During the second reflecting team Dina voiced the concern that Bill might feel picked on by the way we had made space for Pat to express her feelings of inequality. By empowering Pat did we disempower Bill? By asking these questions, we invited Bill to let us know whether we were on a track that suited him. In reflecting on the team's reflections, he said that he didn't feel ganged up on. He assured us that he grew up with four sisters, and he was willing to hear anything we might be thinking regarding men's disrespectful treatment of women. He said he was just glad that Pat was talking: 'She could say anything, I'm just glad to hear her talk'.

In our work since this particular session, Pat, Bill, the team, and I have been able to have open-ended discussions about the broader social context that supports hierarchies and inequalities. We have been able to free up our environment enough to create an area where we could explore the problem of hierarchies in personal and professional relationships. We have developed a more complex understanding of how discourses in those larger realms create closed-off areas where people often fear to tread – an understanding of how labels, fear of not doing it right, and societal silence lead us to collude with the problem.

I believe that narrative therapy's emphasis on questions (instead of answers or so-called truths) is an important factor in our success. Focusing on asking questions rather than giving answers helps us stay grounded in the experience of the people who consult with us. Are our ideas tracking with their ideas? Do they feel comfortable with the direction of the work? Are we getting it right? Are we attending too much to our own agenda? Constantly raising questions such as these produces an environment that allows therapists and the people who consult with them to be mutual catalysts and witnesses of change – a place in which it feels safe for everyone (therapists, too) to try on new ideas, perceptions, and behaviors. We all become members of the same team, supporting each other in the process of change and benefiting from the effects of each other's changes.

We all reflect

We would like to end by providing our thoughts about two questions that readers of this paper might be considering at this point: 'Why should I try to minimize hierarchy in therapy?' and 'Since I don't usually work with a team, how can I minimize hierarchy in my day-to-day work?'

Why Minimize Hierarchy?

- So that the people who consult therapists can feel larger.

  Remember how I (Pat) said that in most previous therapy I felt like a very small person consulting a giant on a pedestal? I feel like a healthier, more competent person when I feel that I am as big as my therapist.

  Both of us (Pat and Bill) believe that things went smoother and faster when we were all working together as a team or family.

- So that therapy will be more comfortable.

  All of us (Pat, Bill, Dina, Michele, David, Jill, and Gene) are much more comfortable in this team atmosphere where everyone's expertise is valued and no one is expected to have all the answers.

- So that lots of different viewpoints can be shared.

  We all agree that being able to view a difficult situation from more than one perceptual position makes it harder to be stuck. The more points of view, the more possible directions we might move. Minimizing hierarchy maximizes the value of each new viewpoint.

- So that everyone's opinion is valued in evaluating the work.

  Remember how I (David) kept going around in circles with Pat before we learned more about how to minimize hierarchy in our relationship?

- So that we can learn to recognize and challenge oppressive hierarchies in the larger culture.

  Through our struggles to work together more collaboratively, I (Michele) am more able to see some of the ways our larger culture supports and fosters undue hierarchy.

  I (Gene) have been struck over and over again at how Pat's efforts to claim more of a voice for herself support and are supported by our efforts as a team to minimize the influence of cultural prescriptions for hierarchy in our teamwork.

- So that we don't reproduce in therapy some of the oppressive politics that may have contributed to people's problems in the first place.

  As White (in Hoyt & Combs 1996) has noted, 'accountability structures' serve to counter such recapitulizations. The structure we have described helped make us (Michele, Dina, David, Jill, and Gene) accountable to Pat and Bill by showing them our process and including them in evaluating it and questioning us.

- So that therapists can stay grounded in the experience of the people who consult with us.

  We (Michele, Dina, Jill, and Gene) all could tell stories similar to the one of how David and Pat stopped going in circles. The therapy process is much more creative when we act on the belief that the ideas of those we consult with are at least as meaningful as our own.

- So that therapists can learn and grow as they work with others.

  We all agree that when therapists think they have to be experts or that professionalism demands that they maintain a distanced authority, their opportunities for growth and learning are severely restrained. Minimizing hierarchy maximizes the space for development as a person.

- So that secrecy, shame, and blame are minimized.

  Remember how free and open I (Dina) could be with Pat and Bill once I knew they had heard me discuss 'excitement' with Jill in the presession? When I thought I had to keep this sort of discussion secret, inside my head, it was embarrassing. It made me feel stiff, distant, and awkward. It feels much better to be transparent about such things.

  We (Pat and Bill) agree. The willingness of team members to talk about their personal struggles in the therapy process helped us to feel valued and respected. Feeling valued and respected helped us become more invested in the therapy process.

- So that neither therapists nor the people who consult them will feel isolated.

  I (Dina) mentioned this in my earlier reflections, and we all agree that maximizing equality and collaboration minimizes isolation.

How can we minimize hierarchy in our day-to-day work?

All the therapists involved in this project agree that working as a team in the structure that has evolved in the Evanston Family Therapy Center training program has helped us to minimize hierarchy in our work without the team. Most of the structures and practices used in the supervision can inspire similar ways of working when there is no team present. We can think out loud at the beginning of a session about the things that might constrain us from being our best selves, thus alerting both ourselves and the people we are working with to these enemies of good therapy. If these constraints start to appear in the session, we have already paved the way for talking about them and dealing with them directly. We can pause at intervals to reflect on what we are hearing and seeing, becoming a one-person reflecting team. After our reflections we can ask the people we are working with to respond, letting us know if what seems remarkable to us is meaningful to them. As we end a particular session, we can ask people to evaluate and deconstruct the session in much the same way that it happens in the team supervision.

We can strive to stay grounded in the experience of those we work with. I (Michele) have found the following questions helpful: Are my ideas tracking with the other people's ideas? Do they feel comfortable with the direction of the work? Am I getting it right? Am I attending too much to my own agenda?

We (Pat and Bill) think that collaborative therapy asks clients to work hard. It may not be for everybody. We spent twice as much time in each therapy session as we were used to spending. Rather than focusing exclusively on our dilemmas, we listened to therapists talk about some of the difficulties they were experiencing as therapists. Personally, we are glad to have put in the extra time and effort – the payoff is well worth it.

Some questions we've found it useful to ask ourselves

In closing, we (Jill and Gene) would like to offer the following list of questions. We have found them helpful in our quest to deemphasize hierarchy in our work both with and without teams. We have included a few blank spaces so that you can collaborate with us in extending the list and personalizing it for yourself. If you would be willing to send us any questions you add, we would be very glad to receive them and to circulate them to other interested people.

- Am I feeling or acting like an expert?
- Are we collaboratively defining problems based on what is problematic in this person's experience?
- Am I making my work as transparent as possible (being forthright, open, and honest about what I'm bringing into the work)?
- Am I checking in about ideas instead of assuming them to be correct?
- Am I contributing to the creation of a context in which everyone involved has a voice in the relationship and the process?
- Am I inviting discussion of differences (not assuming that there is one right way of thinking about things)?
- Whose language is being privileged here? Am I trying to accept and understand this person's linguistic descriptions? If I am offering ideas in my language, why am I doing that? What are the effects of doing that?
- Am I evaluating this person, or am I inviting her or him to evaluate a wide range of things (such as how therapy is going, preferred directions in life, and so on)?

Notes

1. This chapter was originally published in M.F. Hoyt (ed) 1998: *The Handbook of Constructive Therapies: Innovative approaches from leading practitioners.* San Francisco: Jossey-Bass Publishers.
2. A psychiatrist Pat was consulting had said that she would no longer see Pat unless Pat and Bill were in marital therapy. Bill did not want to come, but agreed to try things out for three sessions. Pat did not like it that she had been prescribed couple therapy with an ultimatum by her psychiatrist.
3. When the year-long team supervision program ended, the couple continued meeting with Dina, and Pat continued her ongoing individual therapy relationship with David.

5

Working with 'Mike and Jan'[1]

The ways in which the following chapter is written was once again very much framed by the context in which it was first published. This chapter was written for a textbook in which the story of a couple was offered and then a number of therapists from differing approaches were asked a series of questions about how their work with this particular couple would progress. Under each of the categories in the paper there were many questions. This was quite a difficult task because the questions we were required to answer often involved assumptions that didn't fit with the ways in which we conceptualised our work. We were therefore having to deconstruct the questions in order to answer them. Although challenging, we also found this process of deconstruction very helpful to us in clarifying our own thinking and practice. Others have told us that they have also found it helpful and this is why we have included this paper here.

We also notice on re-reading that we wrote about 'qualities' and 'characteristics' of people and relationships. Although we did not think about these 'qualities' or 'characteristics' as being fixed or essential, the use of this structuralist language is confusing. We would now use different language. Some of the language (e.g. 'case') was put in place by the original editors.

In republishing this article, we have rearranged it somewhat. We have begun with a brief description of narrative therapy (in order to describe our 'treatment model'). We have then inserted the story of Mike and Jan (which was written by Daittilio & Bevilacqua), and then continued on to describe how we would approach working with this particular couple.

Treatment model: Narrative therapy

Narrative therapy, as we use the term, refers to an interrelated set of values, attitudes, stories, and practices that flow from the work of Michel White and David Epston (Freedman & Combs 1996b; Monk, Winslade, Crocket & Epston 1997; White & Epston 1990, 1992; Zimmerman & Dickerson 1996). White and Epston have drawn on the ideas of post-structuralist scholars such as Michel Foucault (1980), Jerome Bruner (1990), and Barbara Myerhoff (1986) to articulate and embody a creative and inspiring approach to therapy. An important idea in narrative therapy is that stories shape our experience. The stories that we enact with each other are not about our lives; they *are* our lives.

Narrative therapists collaborate with people to change their lives by changing their stories. This would be easy work if we could simply construct any story we wanted, tell it, and have it taken up and lived out by the people who consult with us. But it's not that simple. Some stories have more staying power than others. In any culture at any given time, certain stories are much more a part of the fabric of day-to-day reality than are others. We are born into stories, and those stories shape our perceptions of what is possible. However, we don't usually think of the stories we are born into as stories. We think of them as 'reality'. Stories have the power to shape our experience of reality.

The way we see it, the dominant stories in any society are kept in power by richly interconnected networks of language, beliefs, institutions, customs, laws, etc. We call these networks 'discourses' (Hare-Mustin 1994; Madigan 1996), and we think an important part of therapy is making limiting discourses visible so that people have the opportunity to revise their relationships with them. The dominant discourses in any social network determine (and are determined by) what counts as 'knowledge' or 'truth' in that network. The dominant discourses determine who does and does not have access to power. For example, when our founding fathers wrote the phrase 'all men are created equal', the discourses of their day led people to take for granted that 'men' (when applied to the right to vote) meant 'land-owning white males'. It took, among other things, a civil war to change the discourses so that the taken-for-granted meaning of 'men' in relation to the right to vote was 'males of any color, as long as they are U.S. citizens and not in jail'. It took lots more sweat and strife to change the discourses so that 'men' applied to women as well.[2]

A distinguishing feature of narrative work is that we seek to make visible the discourses that support problematic life narratives. We believe that when the partners in a couple decide to consult with a therapist, they are caught up in limiting and unsatisfying stories of themselves, each other, and the world. We believe that those stories are supported by discourses, and that the discourses tend to be invisible (taken for granted). Highlighting the discourses that support a couple's problems makes it possible for the partners to see each other in the light of different discourses. In that light, they can imagine, experience, and live out more satisfying stories of their relationship.

In the day-to-day work of narrative therapy, we start by getting to know people. In an initial interview, we want to hear at least a few things about people's lives outside of the problem – their interests, their living situation, etc. People often begin to tell us about their problems without being asked. If they don't, after a while we might ask a general question like, 'What brought you here?' We listen to their responses as stories. This is a very different mindset from listening for symptoms that will help establish a diagnosis, for surface clues to deep meaning, for self-defeating cognitions, or for 'facts'. We try to understand what is problematic in people's stories, and we search for descriptions of the problem(s) that are 'experience near' (fitting with their vocabulary and worldview, not ours).

We listen with an attitude of not-knowing (Anderson & Goolishian 1992), that is, we cultivate a genuine curiosity about what people will say. We are not trying to lead people toward some predetermined outcome. At the same time – and this can be a tricky balancing act – we don't want to let the dominant discourses in people's worlds predetermine the outcome. With couples, this often means that we must stay aware of gender discourses (Freedman & Combs 1996a; Goldner 1985; Hare-Mustin 1994; Laird 1989) and how they shape each partner's experience and expectations. As we listen, we ask questions that invite people to consider the effects of the problem(s) on their lives and relationships. This combined focus on discourses and the effects of problems tends to bring forth stories of people's struggles with the limiting effects of dominant cultural narratives on their lives. With couples, this can shift each partner's experience from one of struggling with the other person to one of struggling together to overcome problems coming from outside their relationship. Whether this happens or not, this kind of inquiry tends to deconstruct (White 1991) the problematic story, opening space for the perception of 'unique outcomes' (events that would not have been predicted by the problematic story). As unique outcomes are brought forth, we ask questions that invite people to expand or 'thicken' (Geertz 1978) them into memorable, experientially vivid stories.

Stories need listeners as well as tellers. It is through the interpersonal, societal practice of telling and retelling of stories that people's lives can change. For this reason, narrative therapists have developed many ways of working that involve witnessing. We provide space and time for people to reflect on their own narratives as they emerge. Whenever possible, we use reflecting teams (Andersen 1989) or 'outsider-witness groups' (White 1997) to increase the audience for tellings and retellings. As we will illustrate more fully later in this chapter, when working with couples, we often work so that one partner is in a telling mode while the other is in a witnessing mode. There is a rhythmic alternation between telling and listening, between acting and reflecting, that runs through narrative therapy.

When we say, 'telling and retelling', we are speaking of *embodied* expressions. White often quotes Edward Bruner (1986) to emphasize this point:

> *A ritual must be enacted, a myth recited, a narrative told, a novel read, a drama performed, for these enactments, recitals, tellings, readings, and performances are what make the text transformative ... Expressions are constitutive and shaping, not as abstract texts but in the activity that actualizes the text.* (p. 7)

Because we believe that the new stories that emerge in therapy only become transformative as they are enacted outside of the therapy room, we are interested in documenting and circulating the new stories. To facilitate documentation, we sometimes write letters between therapy meetings. In these letters we might reflect on unique outcomes and ask questions that we didn't ask in the session, hoping that this will thicken and extend the knowledge that had begun to emerge there. We might generate formal documents that list important elements of new narratives and, to encourage the circulation of this knowledge, invite people to share these documents with other people in their lives. Another way we might facilitate circulation of alternative stories as they develop is to invite members of people's social networks (friends, co-workers, bosses, teachers, ministers, etc.) to therapy sessions.

Therapist attributes

Many people in the narrative therapy community have noted that the ideas that have come to be known as narrative therapy constitute a worldview, a way of life. We would not think about attributes a therapist should have, but instead whether she situates herself in a way of living that supports collaboration, social justice, and local, situated, context-specific knowledge rather than normative thinking, diagnostic labeling, and generalized (non-contextualized) 'expert' knowledge. This worldview leads to improvisation and creativity and a commitment to confront the discourses that oppress or limit people as they pursue their preferred directions in life. We think that situating ourselves in this worldview is an ongoing process. An important part of that process for us is asking ourselves certain questions.[3]

Here is a representative list of the kinds of questions we ask ourselves:

- Whose language is being privileged here? Am I bringing forth the stories that these people want to tell in their own words, or am I pushing for the stories that I want to hear, told in my jargon?
- Are there dominant stories that are oppressing or limiting these people's lives? Am I inviting awareness of those stories without becoming oppressive myself?
- Am I evaluating these people, or am I inviting them to evaluate things (how therapy is going, the effects of various practices, preferred directions in life, etc.)?
- Who am I viewing as the 'expert' here, myself or the people I am working with?

- Am I working so as to require these people to enter my expert knowledge, or so as to require myself to enter their worlds?
- Is what I am doing dividing and isolating these people, or bringing forth a sense of community and collaboration?
- Am I situating my opinions in my personal experience? Am I being transparent about my context, my values, and my intentions so that these people can evaluate the effects of my biases?
- Do the questions I am asking conserve dominant social practices or propose alternative practices?
- How am I embodying 'professionalism'? Am I more concerned with how I am looking to my professional colleagues or how I am being experienced by the people who are seeking my help?

Introducing Mike and Jan[4]

Introduction and Case Conceptualization
By Louis J. Bevilacqua and Frank M, Dattilio

The following is a case study of a young married couple: Mike and Jan. A brief narrative containing basic information is provided, including data on psychiatric, medical and social history; and history of substance abuse, child abuse, and criminal involvement. A description of the presenting problem and a history of the couple's difficulties will also be explained in detail.

Case study

Jan and Mike are a middle-class Caucasian couple residing in a suburban neighborhood of the Northeast Central States. Jan is a 49-year-old sales associate for a pharmaceutical company. She has been a sales representative with the same company for the past 14 years. Prior to this career, Jan was employed as a receptionist for a dental office and was also working part-time as a salesperson in a major clothing department store. Jan enjoys reading mystery novels and taking care of her animals, which include three horses, two cats, and two birds. Jan has been married to Mike for the past 12 years. They have had no separations to date. They also do not have any children from this union. Jan was married once before for 3 years. Her marriage ended in divorce due to her husband's continued drug abuse and infidelity. There were no children from Jan's previous marriage.

Mike was also married one time prior. His marriage of 1 year ended in divorce due to his drug abuse. There were no children from this union. Mike is 44 and currently employed as a welder/fitter. He acquired this trade while in high school and has maintained various employment in this field for the past 25 years. He has been employed by four different companies overall, the longest period with his present employer, which has been for the past 10 years. Mike enjoys taking care of animals and working on computers.

Mike and Jan met through a mutual friend during a summer outing. They dated only 4 months before deciding to marry. They decided to skip the formalities and were united by a Justice of the Peace in a rather impromptu fashion. They described their courtship as a fun time that they will always remember. While dating, Mike and Jan enjoyed seeing new films, dining out, attending parties, skiing, and taking care of Jan's animals. When they initially met, Mike had relatively few friends. When they would go out together with other couples, Mike and Jan generally socialized with Jan's friends, whom, Mike claims, eventually became his friends as well. Rarely did they socialize with any of Mike's acquaintances.

Psychiatric history

There is no prior history of psychiatric treatment for Mike. He has never been prescribed psychotropic medication, nor has he been hospitalized for any mental health reasons. Mike reports that during his adolescence, his mother received individual treatment for depression after divorcing his father. She was not treated with any medication that he could recall. Mike's brother received individual therapy for 'behavioral problems' as a teenager. His father viewed therapy as something that only 'crazy' people needed and looked upon therapy with disdain. Mike states that he is interested in initiating therapy in order to reduce the tension that exists between himself and Jan, and denies maintaining any of the same type of biases that his father held about therapy.

Jan reports that she received individual therapy for depression approximately 20 years ago after undergoing a hysterectomy. She recalled this as being part of the aftercare plan recommended by her gynecologist. Jan attended approximately 12 sessions and viewed her time in therapy as being very helpful. She has never been prescribed psychotropic medication, nor has anyone in her family. Jan reports that no one in her family, including herself, has ever been hospitalized for mental illness, and is unaware of any psychiatric history with her extended family.

Medical history

Mike has a history of hypertension and elevated cholesterol levels. He inconsistently follows a diet plan to address these two conditions under the care of his family physician. His father had one heart attack, 5 years ago, and is still living. There is a family history of cancer and glaucoma on his mother's side of the family. His mother is currently in good health.

Jan has no current medical problems. There is a family history of cancer and diabetes on both sides of Jan's parents' family. At the age of 29, Jan underwent a hysterectomy as a result of ovarian cancer. Her first reaction to the news of having cancer was devastation. She was scared of dying. She said that, fortunately, her friends and family were very supportive and the surgery was successful. She also reported that having a child was never something that she was really interested in doing, yet the idea of having a hysterectomy bothered her. Jan recounted, 'I did my share of parenting when I was raising my younger brother John. I used to have occasional thoughts of what it might have been like to have a child, but not for the past 12 or 13 years.' Jan said what really helped her was when she met Mike and he expressed his lack of interest in children. This was a big relief to Jan and was one of the characteristics that she found attractive about him.

Social history

Mike is the youngest of two boys. His older brother, 2 years his senior, received part-time special education classes due to weaknesses in reading and math. His brother also had 'behavioral problems' which became a central focus in the family during his upbringing. While growing up, Mike and his older brother Mark were not very close. Mike tended to stay more to himself, while Mark had lots of friends, but tended to get in trouble for not doing his homework and being disrespectful to teachers. Mike was in regular classes and maintained a C average. He recalls not enjoying school very much. In fact, Mike reports that there was never anything he really liked to do.

One of the things his mom always complained of was that Mike rarely finished anything he started. He remembers taking piano lessons and drum lessons, but quitting each one after a few months. He also tried out for a local baseball league, but quit after the second practice. Throughout elementary school, he was often teased for being the biggest kid in his class and for not being very coordinated. Finally, as Mike entered high school, his father made the suggestion that he become involved with football. This altered his reputation with his peers somewhat, and enhanced his social skills. Mike states that he was teased less by the guys, but still felt very uncomfortable and somewhat afraid of females. He dated on and off throughout high school but never maintained any serious female relationship. His mother never approved of any of the girls that he expressed an interest in. He recalls one of his mother's typical responses being, 'Don't get serious, Michael, it will never last.'

Mike describes his parents as being supportive, but to a limited degree. His father attended every one of his football games, and was very lenient in disciplining the children. When Mike had a problem, however, his father's usual curt response was 'Get over it'. Mike's mother was always there to discuss any problems Mike encountered in life, but tended to be very critical of him in general. He said that no matter what problem he was experiencing, his mother always pointed out that it was somehow related to something that Mike did to cause it, This created a great deal of conflictual feelings toward his mother, whom he views as very controlling and maintaining the power in the family.

In describing discipline, Mike reports that his mother set the rules in the house and that everyone was expected to follow them, even his father. Mike remembers one time that the family was having company. His father spilled a drink on the living room carpet and his mom reacted by yelling at his father and calling him a slob in front of the guests. Mike said his father just left the room and walked out of the house. He did not return home until the next day.

The year Mike graduated from high school, he pursued his trade in welding - something that he trained for in vocational classes and has practiced ever since.

That same year Mike's mother filed for divorce after 20 years of marriage, due to her husband's numerous affairs. Mike described his parents' marriage as involving frequent arguments and several separations, Mike was aware of his father's affairs, and believed they were due to his mother's constant 'nagging' and 'put-downs'. When Mike's mother decided on the divorce, his father moved out.

Mike was very surprised and angered by this decision, but never shared his feelings with anyone. Mike rarely saw his father after he moved out, although they did talk over the phone every couple of weeks. He described his mother as becoming more and more critical and demanding of him. Mike said 2 years later, his brother Mark moved out of the house to live with his girlfriend. Mike lived with his mother until he got married for the first time at 29 years of age.

Mike has maintained contact with both of his parents throughout the years. His father never remarried. The year before Mike married his first wife, his mother married her second husband, to whom she has been married for the last 20 years. Mike describes his mother's second marriage as good, and he currently maintains a fairly positive relationship with his stepfather.

Jan is the oldest of two children. Despite being 5 years his senior, Jan reports a close relationship with her brother, John, during their upbringing. Her parents both had careers, and had little time for Jan and her brother during their childhood. She describes her parents as very lenient and supportive in a remote sort of way. Her parents rarely denied her anything, and frequently bought her and her brother whatever they wanted. Her parents placed a great deal of responsibility on Jan, since she was 5 years older than John. As a result, Jan spent a large portion of her childhood as a caregiver to John. She recalls that often, after school, she would make a snack for her and her brother before they began their homework. Sometimes when her mother was running late, Jan would make dinner for the entire family. She reports having enjoyed this type of responsibility until John started high school and became involved with drugs. Jan had been experimenting with marijuana herself, but saw her brother's use as extensive and clearly destructive. This led to frequent heated arguments between herself and her brother. Her parents were quite liberal regarding the drug use, and saw experimentation as 'normal'. Jan remembers one time that she was expressing her concerns of John's drug use to her parents. Her parents responded by saying, 'As long as he only smokes it on the weekends, we don't think he has a problem'.

Throughout high school, Jan did well academically, and had a number of friends. She reports that her friends were her 'real supports'. Anytime she had a problem, it was her friends who she went to. After graduation, Jan attended college and received a bachelor's degree in philosophy, with a minor in marketing. Upon graduating from college, Jan began working full-time in a local clothing department store.

Substance abuse history

Throughout his senior year in high school, Mike drank alcohol quite heavily on the weekends. At the age of 20, he was introduced to marijuana by a co-worker. His alcohol and marijuana use continued on and off for approximately 10 years. At one point during this time, Mike lost his job as a result of coming to work late and frequently hung-over. Unfortunately, his dismissal did not change his frequency or quantity of substance use, which continued. This did not change until Mike became involved in an auto accident due to his drug use. After running over and killing a dog, he crashed into a telephone pole, totally destroying his car. He was charged with driving under the influence and spent one night in jail. This also resulted in Mike's dismissal from his second job. That same year, Mike's first wife divorced him.

At that point, Mike began thinking that his drug use was becoming out of control. He decided to stop using all substances except alcohol. This lasted for 3 years, until one day a co-worker offered Mike some marijuana after work and he accepted it. He explained this relapse as a result of stress from work. In particular, Mike described experiencing difficulty getting along with a female co-worker with whom he was competing for a position. Mike claims that the last straw to this conflict was when his co-worker was finally chosen for this position over him and received a substantial raise. Mike believed that she was underqualified for this position, and consequently he resigned from his position 2 weeks later.

Mike continued to use alcohol and marijuana for another 10 years. One night, after using alcohol rather heavily, Mike was driving home from a friend's house when he passed out and remained unconscious for several hours. When he awoke, Mike realized that he was in the middle of a cornfield and could not remember how he got there. Following this blackout period, Mike went through a 28-day in-patient drug and alcohol treatment program. As a result he has been substance-free for the last 7 months, and has also been attending Narcotics Anonymous meetings on a weekly basis.

Jan experimented with marijuana and alcohol while in high school and college. After graduating from college, she stopped using controlled substances, except for an occasional glass of wine. During her first marriage, she began using marijuana again. She and her first husband used together frequently. One year prior to separating from her first husband, Jan stopped using and began attending Narcotics Anonymous meetings.

Child abuse

Mike was sexually molested between the ages of 7 and 9 by a paternal aunt. This involved her fondling and kissing Mike on a sporadic basis. He reports that this ended when his aunt moved away. He has not disclosed this information to anyone besides his wife, Jan, and the therapist.

Jan reports no history of any type of child physical or sexual abuse.

Criminal history

Mike was arrested for driving while under the influence and spent one night in jail. His license was suspended for 6 months. Jan has no criminal history.

Presenting problem

Jan made the initial call for an appointment for marital therapy. She stated that she and her husband were experiencing difficulty achieving emotional intimacy due to continual conflicts and lack of effective resolutions. Jan and Mike tend to avoid discussing conflicts with each other. When they do argue, Jan tends to criticize Mike, and he simply dismisses what Jan says as being trivial. At times, Mike will avoid being around the house, particularly when Jan is at home. He does this to avoid tension in the relationship. This conflict-avoidance pattern of interacting has led to a lack of trust and emotional distance between them, which has naturally affected their intimacy. There have been times when attending therapy was discussed, but neither followed through due to periodic improvements.

For the past 7 months, Jan and Mike reported, they were getting along fairly well. Mike was calling Jan and letting her know where he was and what time he was coming home. Jan felt that she had begun to trust Mike again. This trust was violated, however, when 2 weeks prior Mike came home at 2:30 AM. Mike said he went to Jennifer's house for a party. Jennifer has been a family friend for the past 20 years and the party was for those who helped her to relocate to her new residence. Jan did not want to go to the party and secretly wished that Mike would decline as well. Unfortunately, she never told Mike her true feelings, and Mike ended up going by himself. Mike said he had fallen asleep while at Jennifer's home and did not wake up until 1:00 AM. Jennifer lives an hour and a half away and Mike said that he drove straight home when he realized what had happened. Jan felt that Mike should have called her immediately and had erred in his judgement. Mike said he just wanted to get home as fast as he could, and knew in advance that Jan would be upset. This incident resulted in a heated argument, that included a discussion about divorce. Jan told Mike she was not willing to continue the relationship because she didn't feel as though she could trust him any longer. Mike felt this was totally unfair of Jan. Mike pointed out to Jan that in the last 6 weeks he has done everything he said he would and that Jan should still be able to trust him. Despite Mike's efforts, Jan said she still wanted to pursue a divorce. Mike angrily responded by saying, 'Fine, if you want a divorce, go for it. Let's do it tomorrow.' The next day Jan reconsidered her position and apologized to Mike, but did admit that she was confused about her feelings. Mike acknowledged Jan's confusion and admitted to his own frustrations with the marriage. It was at that point that Jan suggested they begin couples therapy, and Mike agreed.

History of presenting problem

Throughout the marriage, Mike and Jan have avoided discussing any conflicts, and do not recall ever really resolving any of their disagreements completely. Usually, arguments would end with Mike leaving the house for several hours. When they would reconvene, they would avoid bringing up the issue of contention, and the matter would simply be dropped. The majority of their arguments involved Jan's complaints about Mike's being undependable, and especially concerning his drug abuse. Mike would rationalize that he continued to use substances because of Jan's 'nagging'. Whenever there would be disagreements, Mike would tell Jan to 'just drop it'. This tended to infuriate Jan, and she would yell and cry more profusely. Eventually, Mike would leave the room and, sometimes, the house. Unfortunately, the matters would never be resolved – and would only be tucked away until they resurfaced in another argument and continued to erode the relationship.

Critical life events timeline

1948	-	Jan is born
1951	-	Mike's brother, Mark is born
	-	Mike's parents are married
1953	-	Mike is born
	-	Jan's brother, John is born
1966	-	Jan graduates high school
1970	-	Jan graduates college – B.A. in Philosophy
	-	Jan begins working at a clothing department store
1971	-	Mike graduates high school
	-	Mike's parents divorce
1973	-	Mark moves out of his mother's home
	-	Mike begins using marijuana
1977	-	Jan is diagnosed with cancer and has a hysterectomy
	-	Jan attends 12 sessions of therapy for depression
1980	-	Jan marries her first husband
1981	-	Mike's mother remarries

1982	-	Mike gets married for the first time
	-	Jan stops using marijuana and starts attending Narcotics Anonymous
1983	-	Mike is charged with a D.U.I, and loses his second job
	-	Jan divorces her first husband
	-	Mike separates from his first wife
1984	-	Mike and Jan meet through a mutual friend
1985	-	Mike and Jan get married
1986	-	Mike begins using marijuana again
	-	Mike quits his job
1987	-	Mike starts working at his fourth and current job
1997	-	Mike attends inpatient drug and alcohol treatment program
	-	Mike starts attending Narcotics Anonymous meetings
	-	Mike and Jan begin couples therapy

A narrative response to the story of Mike and Jan

Assessment

Two ideas that inform narrative work seem particularly relevant in responding to this category and set of questions. The first is 'the interpretive turn' (J. Bruner 1986), which supports the idea that people are in a better position to interpret their own experience than outsiders are. In keeping with this idea, as stated in the previous sections, we encourage those with whom we work to be in an evaluative position about the work and about their experience. Insofar as possible, we avoid the position of making professional, 'knowing', assessments. Because we are interested in detailed, context-specific narratives, we shy away from standardized instruments and psychological testing.

The second idea is that we think about information as being *generated,* rather than 'gathered' in therapeutic conversations. In a rather literal way, we believe that we are making ourselves and each other up as we go along. This is a poststructuralist idea. We do not assume that a couple has a particular interactional or relational structure that we can assess. We do not think of people or relationships as having stable, quantifiable identities or 'typical' characteristics, so we do not try to uncover or gather information about such characteristics. Instead, we think of people's lives as being multistoried, and we believe that each new telling generates new possibilities for interpretation and action.

We would be interested in asking questions that would invite Jan and Mike to tell more satisfying and useful stories of their relationship. As these stories took shape, we would invite them to assess their usefulness. We would want to know whether the new stories spoke to them of a more satisfying identity as a couple. In telling these stories and reflecting on them, Jan and Mike would be collaborating with us in an ongoing assessment of the new expressions of themselves and their relationship.

Here are some questions we might ask in eliciting Jan's and Mike's assessments:

- What name would you give the problem?
- What is it like to have the experience of the problem?
- What effect does the problem have on your life?
- What effect does the problem have on your relationship with each other?
- What effect does the problem have on other relationships?
- How does the problem affect your relationship with yourself?
- Is this what you want for your relationship? Why or why not?
- Is this what you want for yourself? Why or why not?
- Are we talking about what you want to be talking about?
- Is this conversation useful?
- How is it useful?

While we favor leaving assessment in the hands of the people who consult with us, it would be misleading to imply that we make no assessments of any kind. Rachel Hare-Mustin (1994) makes the argument that if we simply reflect what our clients say in therapy, nothing new will happen. We see it as our responsibility to bring in new discourses. One kind of assessment, then, that we make has to do with which parts of Jan and Mike's story might be located in discourses that are invisible to them. We would be interested in asking questions to locate their problems in such discourses and to give Jan and Mike an opportunity to decide (in this way leaving 'assessment' as much as possible still in their hands) where they stand and where they would like their relationship to be in the face of such discourses. Because each question leads to the next in ways that none of us can know until they are spoken, it is quite difficult to describe exactly how this might go. However, we might initiate such a conversation with some of the following questions:

- In the pattern you describe of avoiding conflict, part of the description included a reference to Jan 'nagging'. Do you think that description of nagging is more often applied to men or women?
- *(If the answer is 'women')* Do you think there is a comparable way of relating that men would be described as using? What would that be called?
- What do you think supports women and men trying to influence each other in such different ways?

Case conceptualization

The worldview that we subscribe to influences how we read the material in the case presentation. Within our worldview, we do not think of the material as descriptions of or clues to personality. Within that worldview, we are not looking for healthy or unhealthy behavior, normal or abnormal affective states, rational or irrational cognitions. We are not making global assessments of Jan's and Mike's functioning. Instead, we read the material as stories which are expressions of Jan's and Mike's experience. In working with them we would remain steadfast in our belief that other experiences could be storied, and that these other stories would speak differently of their lives and identities. We would consider it part of our task not to let the problem-filled stories dominate our view of Jan and Mike or of their relationship.

As we described in our answer to the question about assessment, we would hope to find ways for Jan and Mike to be doing any evaluating that was done.

In keeping with that stand, we would want to know how Mike and Jan might describe their desired directions in life in relation to the problems that beset them, both individually and as a couple. We would be looking for sparkling moments – events in their stories that would not have been predicted by the problem-filled stories that have brought them to therapy.

For example, if they had named the pattern of avoiding conflict as a problem which has brought distrust, emotional distance, avoidance, criticism, and tension into their lives, we would be listening for moments that seem to stand outside of the stories of conflict avoidance and its effects. As we heard about events that sounded like such moments, we would ask questions about them. Here are some of the questions we might ask:

- You have described your courtship as a fun time you will always remember. When you think about it what stands out for you?
- What do you notice in your partner that the distrust and tension may have kept you from seeing lately? What do you see about your relationship?
- We are interested to hear that although you have talked about therapy before from time to time, you did not follow through because things got better. Can you tell us about this getting better? What did each of you contribute to it? How did it happen? Was there preparation involved or did you simply find yourselves doing things differently? How would you explain that?
- As you hear your partner describe his or her part in things getting better, what does it tell you about his or her motivation and intentions in the relationship? Is that something that you already knew about? If so, how did you know it?
- You've told us that for the past 7 months you have been getting along fairly well. Could you describe a typical evening or Saturday during that time of getting along well? When you look at that, what do you learn about your relationship and about each other?
- Can you see moments during that evening or Saturday when you could have been derailed by the pattern of avoiding conflict, but you weren't?
- What went into keeping your relationship the way you wanted it instead of the way the pattern of conflict-avoidance might have wanted it? What can you see that your partner contributed to that happening? How would you name that quality in your partner?

We might also ask similar kinds of questions about Jan's and Mike's individual stories.

Through questions of this kind, we might develop a list of events that would not have been predicted by the stories of conflict avoidance, distrust, emotional distance, criticism, and tension. Each of these events, pending Jan and Mike's confirmation, would be a candidate for 'unique outcome' status. To build on these unique outcomes in the treatment process, we would ask questions that invited the telling and retelling of stories having to do with them. As such stories were told, we would hear descriptions of qualities or characteristics in the relationship and in each partner that were not part of the pattern of avoiding conflict.

Hypothetically, let's suppose that the couple named 'commitment' and 'closeness' as qualities of their relationship that emerged in these stories, and that they named 'warmth' and 'understanding' as qualities that Jan showed and 'strength' and 'fun-loving' as qualities that Mike showed.

To thicken the stories of these qualities, we might ask questions such as the following:

- Have there been other times that you have seen the commitment and closeness in your relationship?
- Can you tell us about these times?
- What do these experiences mean to you?
- If you held these memories close to you in your heart and mind at some of the times that the conflict avoidance pattern (or distrust, etc.) tends to take over, how would that make a difference?

To Jan:

- Do you like being described as understanding and warm?
- Why do you like that?
- Who from your past do you think would have noticed these qualities in you at a very early age?
- What would they have observed?

To Mike:

- What is it like hearing Jan's memory of that?
- Does it put the story you told about the 'nagging' in a different light? How?
- Which of those ways of looking at it do you prefer? Why?

- Do you often think of yourself as fun and strong?
- In which contexts do you think those aspects of yourself are most at play?
- What do you think it would be like if Jan had more experience of you the way you are in those contexts?

To Jan:

- What do you think it would be like if you were more in on the way Mike is in those contexts?

To Mike:

- If you were going to create that context more at home, what would be your first step?

Treatment goals

A general goal for our work is to help the members of couples experience themselves as living out preferred stories of themselves and their relationships. Because we strive to conduct our conversations in the realm of the not-yet-spoken, we do not set goals at the outset with the couples we see. We listen for sparkling moments or hidden presences that would not have been predicted by the problematic story. When we hear what sounds to us like such moments, we ask questions about them to see if they might be openings to new stories. None of us know where these stories will take us.

We speak of 'projects' or 'directions in life' more often than we speak of goals. We believe that this language leaves more room for revision and redecision along the way. It fits better with the 'making it up as we go along' atmosphere that we value. Projects are usually identified and named in relation to problems. If Jan and Mike had named the problem 'the conflict-avoiding pattern', or 'distrust', or 'tension', they might name the project 'closeness', 'strength', or 'warmth'. The names emerge through the telling of counterstories to the problem.

In the course of therapy, we would often ask Jan and Mike to make evaluations of how things are going in terms of the problem and the project. They may come in and tell about something that happened since they last met and we might say, 'Is that way of being more on the side of avoiding conflict or more on the side of closeness?' In this way they continually evaluate their experience in terms of the problem and the project.

While we would not set goals for Jan and Mike based on our ideas of how a couple should be, or on any established norms, or ideas of 'health', we would not say that we think all stories are equal. We take strong stands against (for example) oppression, violence, and exploitation, and we strive to be transparent about our own values and biases. Even in taking a strong stand against something, we would seek Jan and Mike's collaboration.

Techniques and interventions

Because we place such a high premium on collaboration and avoidance of 'expert' knowledge, we prefer not to use words like 'techniques' or 'interventions'. We speak instead of 'practices'. While certain practices are widely used and perhaps even characteristic of narrative therapy, we would not want anyone to use these practices in a rote or standardized way. That said, it is very likely that we would use questions, transparency, externalizing conversations, developing a history of the present, some reflective practices, and taking-it-back practices in working with Jan and Mike. We might also use an outsider witness group or reflecting team, letter writing, documents, and internalized other questioning.

Questions

We would strive to do most of the interview through questions. We find that questions help construct a collaborative atmosphere. There are not particular questions that we would use or decide upon beforehand outside of the conversation. We would propose a domain through a question and Jan or Mike's response would further the story within that domain. We will sketch an idealized map here, emphasizing that there is not a particular sequence to how we would do this work. It would evolve in conversation with Mike and Jan.

We would begin the interview by asking questions of both Mike and Jan, to get to know them as people – not in terms of the problems that brought them. They might fill us in on their work or some of the interests mentioned in the case material or anything else of interest to them. This initial conversation would be important in communicating our understanding that their identities include much more than the problems that brought them.

Transparency

We would then invite them to ask us any questions. Our interest in putting forward this invitation would be to minimize the power differential inherent in client-therapist relationships. For many people, this invitation signals that the context of working in this way may be 'different' than other therapies. It would offer us the opportunity to begin the practice of transparency – making our biases and ideas visible and traceable to particular experience, rather than representing the voice of family therapy or professional discourse. We think that practices of transparency, which would continue throughout the work, would help the couple know how to take our ideas. At this same point, especially with a heterosexual couple, we might introduce a conversation about gender, especially if only one of us were working with Jan and Mike. In that case, we would want to mention that our own gender would make it more likely that we understand one of their experiences more fully than the other's.

Externalizing conversations

After we had gotten to know each other a bit, we would be interested in having a conversation about the problem. We would hope to engage in a deconstructive, externalizing conversation in which we asked Mike and Jan to name problems (these could be different problems for each of them or a shared problem). We would have at least three ideas in mind: first, to separate Jan and Mike from the problem by speaking about it in an externalized way; second, to unmask what contributes to and supports the problem; and third, to note the effects of the problem on their lives, relationships, and identities (both as a couple and individually).

In the second purpose we mentioned – to unmask with them what contributes to and supports the problem – we would be wondering about power. With both heterosexual and same-sex couples, we wonder if gender and cultural specifications play a role in power inequities. With Jan and Mike, we wonder, for example, if gender specifications may be intertwined with some social class differences. Specifically, the material indicates that Jan graduated from college and Mike began working straight out of high school. Jan works as a sales associate for a pharmaceutical company and Mike works as a welder/fitter. We might ask about whether Jan earns more money and if she does, what the effects of that have been for this couple. In our culture, the traditional expectations are that men should be more responsible as wage-earners and that as 'the head of the family' men should have greater qualifications, such as more education. If there is a discrepancy in earning, we would wonder if the cultural expectations have created problems for this couple around the meaning of their different salaries. We would also wonder about the different status and symbols of status involved in each of their jobs and levels of education and how those interact with gender specifications. We would explore this area through many questions, following their experience. Our intention would be to expose the role that cultural specifications play, so that this couple could consider whether the problems are lodged in those specifications, rather than in each other.

As problems are named and externalized and their effects are mapped out, we would be listening for hidden presences – sparkling moments whose existence would not be predicted by the problematic stories. We would view these sparkling moments or unique outcomes as possible entry ways to alternative stories. Through questions, we would invite Jan and Mike to thicken the stories of experiences that stand outside of the problems. As these stories developed, we would ask them to evaluate whether these stories fit with their preferences in life. For example, the material indicates that Jan is 49 and that Mike is 44. In our culture, the normative story is that in heterosexual relationships the man is older. Somehow this couple made up their own mind instead of letting cultural specifications come between them in regard to age. We would be interested in the story of this, and particularly in what good things it says about them as a couple.

We would think about this process as the deconstruction of problematic stories and development of preferred stories. As preferred stories are told and retold, we would expect that they would speak to Jan and Mike of preferred directions and possibilities for their relationship and their identities within it.

Developing a history of the present

As new stories develop we would be interested in developing their roots. This has also been referred to as mapping a 'history of the present'. For example, it might emerge that one of the ways that Mike has turned his back on drugs for the last 7 months has been through telling himself how important this is to Jan. Jan, in reflecting on this new aspect of the story, might name the quality this shows in Mike as 'loyalty'. To develop a history of the present, we might begin to ask Mike if he could tell other stories in which his loyalty really showed.

In response to our questions, Mike might tell of his devotion to a high school friend who was badly injured in an accident – how he had helped him with his homework, driven him to school, and visited him during extended stays in the hospital. He might then talk about how, later on in their lives, he risked his own job to help the friend find work. Jan would hear these stories from a witnessing, reflective position and they might remind her of other times in which Mike's loyalty has been evident. We could ask her questions to bring forth thick descriptions of those stories.

This whole conversation would invite both partners to step into a world where Mike is a loyal person and has been a loyal person for a long time. In that world, their relationship might feel more full of good possibilities. This is just a tiny example of how alternative stories could be developed that the couple could then decide if they preferred.

Reflecting Practices

We would expect Jan and Mike to have different stories about the same events in their relationship, just as we would expect each of them to name different events in their relationship as especially significant. These differences often lead to conflict. Many couples approach therapy as a venue where only one version of the truth can prevail. Some people interrupt their partner to argue or correct. Others keep track of the errors they hear so that they can set the therapist straight. Others are intent on explaining how they see the situation their partner is describing differently. These common practices get in the way of each person really witnessing or even hearing his or her partner's story.

We would structure much of the work by speaking directly with either Jan or Mike and asking the other to be in a listening position. At intervals, we would switch and ask the listener to reflect on what he or she heard. Much of our work with couples involves this practice of speaking with one member at a time and then turning to the other to ask for reflections. In this atmosphere, with our questions facilitating, the person in the 'witnessing' position often understands his or her partner in ways that are relatively free of defensiveness, argumentation, and competition.

Taking-it-back practices

We find that invariably in our work with couples we gain something. We hope that we always include taking-it-back practices in our work. These consist of finding respectful ways to let the people we work with know that the conversations they have included us in have given something to us. We would 'take it back' by acknowledging to Jan and Mike what the work with them means to us. We might do this by telling how some step they had taken together had given us the courage to take a risky step in our own lives. Or we might share how something we had learned in working with them had been useful in our work with another couple.

Other practices

There are other practices that we might use in working with Jan and Mike. An *outsider witness group* or *reflecting team* who could witness the couple's new, preferred, stories and participate in the definitional ceremony {Meyerhoff 1986) of telling and retelling them would be additive. Also, we might collaborate with Jan and Mike to create *letters* and *documents* (White & Epston 1990) to thicken and document their preferred stories and stands on life. Additionally, some of the conversations might make use of internalized other interviewing (Epston 1993; MacCormack & Tomm 1998) in which we would ask questions of the internalized Jan in Mike and the internalized Mike in Jan.

Pitfalls

We would not anticipate pitfalls, just as we would not be able to anticipate what will be the preferred stories that Jan and Mike author over the course of the therapy. In general, when things were not going in a direction that Jan and Mike clearly preferred, we would think again about deconstructing problematic stories. Perhaps the problem as Jan and Mike first named it was 'distrust' and the project was 'closeness'. If, after a time of moving in the direction of more closeness, they come in complaining of being distant from each other, we would wonder what is getting in the way of closeness now. Perhaps distrust has taken over again. Perhaps we haven't facilitated the telling and retelling of closeness stories enough, or thickened and circulated the stories enough, for them to have become a dependable part of Jan and Mike's reality. Maybe what is getting in the way is no longer distrust. Perhaps the drug culture has gotten a grip on Mike again.[5] If the drug culture was what was getting in the way of closeness now, we would inquire about its effects on Mike and Jan and on their relationship. In the course of this inquiry, we would be on the lookout for unique outcomes and preferred directions in life. As they emerged, we would seek thick, memorable, widely circulated stories of them.

It is difficult for us to say how we might address boundaries or limits with Mike and Jan. As we have already stated, we are clearly and outspokenly against violence, oppression, and exploitation. We think more in these terms than we do in terms of 'boundaries' or 'limits'. To us, the discourse of separation and individuation has been overly valued, and these terms derive from that discourse. We would be interested in finding ways for Mike and Jan to consider their relationship in the light of discourses that support collaboration, connection, and interdependence.

Areas to avoid

There are no areas that we would want to avoid addressing with Mike and Jan.

Inclusion of other family members

Since ours is a social constructionist therapy, we value community. We are always on the lookout for other people to participate in the tellings and retellings of people's preferred stories. Cultivating an audience for new stories can thicken them and create a support system for them. At the very least we would include other people through inquiring about them and their viewpoints in our conversations with Jan and Mike. We would ask them questions that include other people, such as the following:

- Who would have predicted this step you are taking?
- What do they know about your relationship that would have led them to predict this?
- If I were to interview them, what memory might they tell me about that fits with this step?
- What words would they use to describe this quality in your relationship?
- Would it be helpful to hold this person's view of your relationship closer?

We would also be interested in having other people actually join our sessions. This could be in the form of an outsider witness group or reflecting team, if Jan and Mike were agreeable and if that fit with the therapy context.

With the couple's permission, we might ask others who might be part of a supporting community, whether or not they are family members, to join us. It would emerge in conversation who might be relevant to invite. For example, if the problem is named as 'distrust', the drug culture might have played a big role in luring Mike away from closeness and in alienating Jan. This distance and alienation might have been identified as contributing to the distrust. If the couple has a friend who has successfully walked away from drugs and has supported this couple in staying away from drugs, it might be appropriate to invite that friend as a witness who could reflect on the stories that came forth in therapy. Mike's AA sponsor might be a possibility.

Another way we might include other people would be to initiate a letter-writing campaign. We might ask friends, relatives, and associates, often people from different periods and places in Mike's and Jan's lives, to send letters about their experience of that person.

We would certainly, with Mike and Jan's permission, be interested in including other involved professionals. In the work of deconstructing problematic stories and authoring preferred ones, we are very interested in facilitating community inclusion and support for preferred stories. As we talked with other professionals, we would be interested in circulating alternative strands of story that we hoped would become part of their way of relating to Jan and Mike. Their involvement in the therapy process would be negotiated, first with Jan and Mike and then with each particular professional person.

Homework

Our associations to 'homework' and 'assignments' are hierarchical. When we use these words, we imagine one person telling the others what to do (and usually when and how to do it). Since we are interested in contributing to a collaborative context that minimizes hierarchy, we would not choose to use these metaphors. However, an implication in the idea of homework is that things happen outside of the therapy room that contribute to the process. That idea is very much a part of our work.

Lynn Hoffman (1990) writes that in moving into a social constructionist way of working it is not that she doesn't do what she did before, she just does it more tentatively. If, in the developing of a preferred story in therapy, either Jan or Mike had the idea of doing something in keeping with that story – or if we had a thought of something they might do – we might (tentatively) wonder what it would be like to actually do it. For example, if we were developing stories of trust, and Jan and Mike told us about long, sharing conversations that contributed to trust they used to have while eating out together during their courtship, we might wonder if that would be something they would be interested in doing again. If they decide to follow through on this, it would probably have something in common with doing a homework assignment.

Our hope is that in the telling and retelling of preferred stories, Jan and Mike would begin to live out the preferred stories, rather than the ones that they find problematic. We would hope that between meetings they would be doing things and thinking in ways that would be in keeping with their preferred stories., One thing that we might do to aid in this process is write letters summarizing preferred stories as they are developing and asking questions that might contribute to the further development of those stories. Or we might send a document summarizing the stand they decided to take in relationship to the problem. Most couples who receive such letters or documents in the mail tell us that they read and reread them, sometimes posting them, and sometimes carrying them around to consult with when problems seem to be on the verge of making a comeback.

Here is a letter that we might send, based simply on the information supplied. Since we would ask different questions if we had interviewed the couple ourselves, our letter would be somewhat different and would probably include a brief summary of our understanding of the couple's stories.

Dear Jan and Mike,

We enjoyed getting to know you a bit at our first meeting. We are sending this letter simply to raise a few questions that occurred to us after you left. If you would like, we can talk about them next time.

One part of the interview that stayed with us was your comment that for the last 7 months, with the exception of the event that led to your coming here, you have been getting along fairly well. We would be interested in what getting along fairly well means to each of you. What kinds of things are different? What would you each say that your partner contributes to the difference? What are you each aware of contributing? If you could tell us about a particular time that was characteristic of getting along, what would you tell us about? What do you think it says about your potential as a couple that you could get along fairly well for 7 months? Did each of you do things in the months prior to the 7 months that laid the groundwork for this time?

If we understood you correctly, one important characteristic of your relationship during this time was trust. The trust seemed to be in danger when Mike came home at 2:30 AM without calling. Within a day, you as a couple came together and decided to begin couples therapy. Do you think that that says something about your motivation to keep trust in your relationship?

We also noted that Mike has been substance-free for 7 months. Is there a connection between your getting along and the elimination of drugs? The correlation leads us to wonder if the drugs came between you or got in the way of your being able to see what might be possible. Does that fit for you? If it does, now that drugs aren't blurring your vision, what do you see in your relationship that drugs had obscured?

Another thing we noticed, Jan, probably because we both enjoy reading mysteries, is that you are a mystery reader too. You know how a good mystery has clues leading up to its resolution? We were just wondering if there are clues in your life together that point in the direction of how you would like things to be.

If any of our thoughts or questions are of interest to you, we would be happy to talk about them together.

'Til next time,
Jill and Gene

Even if no ideas were suggested and no letters were sent, we would expect that things would happen between meetings that could contribute to alternative stories. We might begin a therapy conversation with Mike and Jan by reading our notes from the previous conversation. The notes would summarize the developing stories, and we could then ask the couple what has happened since our last conversation that would extend these stories. They can then reflect on the time between meetings in relation to the stand they have taken and the preferences for their lives and relationship that they have named in previous therapy conversations.

Timeline for therapy

At the end of each meeting, we would ask Jan and Mike if the interview was helpful and if so, how it was helpful. Then we would ask if they wanted to come back and if so, when they wanted to come back. For most people, this is an unexpected way of negotiating timing. We do it this way because we want to privilege the experience and wisdom of the people we work with, rather than our own.

Some couples find our asking them about the timing confusing. They may ask how often we *usually* see people. We generally say something like the following: 'You have decided that you want to do something about a problem and we see ourselves as consultants in that project. How often you want to consult us really is your choice. Some people have told us it works best for them if it is often enough to keep them organized and reminded of the work they are engaged in, and not so often that they haven't had time to reflect on the last interview and to try out any ideas they have had. Different couples have different schedules and different amounts of time available to them, so we don't know what would be most fitting for you.'

Other couples are delighted to hear that they don't have to come every week. Some may want to come more frequently at times of intense difficulty and less frequently as they become more securely situated in preferred stories.

How long the therapy extends over time would again be up to Jan and Mike. Some couples name a problem, begin to develop preferred stories, and experience themselves as being 'over a hump' in just a few meetings. They may end therapy for good or they may come back at times they feel stuck. Other couples value having a format where they can reflect on their ongoing experience. Over the course of therapy, they may name a number of different problems and develop many rich strands of story. They value having witnesses and a time they can set aside for this process.

We would be flexible about whether and when to see either Mike or Jan individually. If Jan came to an appointment greeting us by saying, 'Mike called me on his way here. He couldn't leave his job so we decided I'd come alone', we would see her alone. We might well write a letter to Mike filling him in on the conversation and asking some questions about what he would have contributed if he had been there. We would see either Mike or Jan individually by plan if they requested it. In such instances, the other would also have the opportunity to be seen alone.

If either Mike or Jan was asking to be seen alone because they thought a particular problem was 'theirs', we would wonder if it might be useful to have the other as a witness. Although we would try to be flexible, one thing we would think about and perhaps talk with Mike and Jan about is the possibility that we might become more involved in the stories we heard from the couple member we were seeing alone rather than being equally immersed in both of their stories. That would be a reason to confer with them about a possible referral to someone else for individual therapy. Another reason would be if one of them was interested in talking about something they both agreed was separate from their relationship and not important to work with together, for example, something having to do with work.

Termination and relapse prevention

Since we would be thinking of ourselves as consultants to Jan and Mike, they would have more say in when and how the consultation ended than we would. People make only one appointment at a time with us. They don't have a regular appointment time unless their schedules demand it. At the end of each time, we ask if they would like to come back and if so, when. There would come a time when Mike and Jan would decide not to come back. Most likely they would realize that they were nearing the end of the process and tell us that a few sessions before they actually stopped. We feel most satisfied if therapy ends with people living out stories that they prefer. We are more certain that this is the case when those stories have been told and retold in the consulting room and contrasted with the way things were before. If a couple suddenly and unexpectedly feels 'done', we might suggest another meeting to look at how far they've come, and what it means about them as a couple that they have been able to do this work together.

We do know that Jan and Mike would have the final say in when therapy ended, but we don't know where this work would lead them and what stories would unfold as they began taking the problems apart.

Although therapy with Mike and Jan would end, our relationship with them would not necessarily end. We might ask them if they would be willing to serve as consultants to us about a particular problem that they had conquered. They could do this by being interviewed to make a consultation tape that we might show to other couples facing similar problems, or we might ask if they would be willing to come back and serve as outsider witnesses on a reflecting team for people struggling with problems similar to the ones they had overcome.

Notes

1. Combs, G. & Freedman, J. 2000: 'Narrative therapy with couples.' In Dattilio, F.M. & Bevilacqua, L. (eds), *Comparative Treatments for Relationship Dysfunction.* New York: Springer.
2. We heard this example in a snippet of a radio interview with a Derrida scholar, whose name we did not hear.
3. The original questions on this list came to us in a personal communication from David Epston, who said that he and Michael White had developed them for themselves. Over the years, we have revised the list and added questions of our own.
4. Jan and Mike are a real couple whose names and identity have been changed significantly to protect their true identity.
5. We do not mean to imply here that we would not have talked with them about the drug culture until this point in therapy. We may well have asked about it, but perhaps they thought at the time that that particular problem was behind them.

PART TWO

Some ideas for working with children

In this section we have included two papers that describe some of our adventures in working with children. While work with young people is not a major part of our work, it is an area which we delight in when the opportunities arise. These two papers are by no means exhaustive descriptions of ways of working with children. In fact, they are just the opposite. We have simply included here some stories of work and ideas that we have found helpful in our consultations with children.

6

Witnessing bravery: Narrative ideas for working with children and families[1]

by

Virginia Simons[2] & Jill Freedman

This paper was created from a collaboration between Virginia (Jenny) Simons and me (JF). Virginia shared office space with us for a number of years and during that time she worked primarily with young children. In those days, our lives and work were constantly enriched by these children's laughter, voices and stories. Every day or so, some small person would stop us and say 'do you know what I did?' and we would be introduced to some of the sparkling moments of their lives. Jenny would also come and invite us to be a part of various celebrations and rituals in which documents would be read and congratulations offered. We'd be given a hat and a piece of cake and we'd just love being there. We hope this spirit of delight is conveyed in the following pages.

The Barry Levinson film *Avalon* portrays the overlapping worlds of adults and children in an extended family. At one point Michael's father tells him: 'When I was just a little younger than you, I thought the world was made up of just big people and little people. What I couldn't understand is why everything was made for the big people; the chairs and tables were too big, the sinks were too high, even the toilet bowl was too big.'

Later in the film, after he fails to heed a warning to stop playing with matches, Michael frantically stomps the flames of a fire he and his cousin have set in the basement of his father's new store. After believing they have stifled the flames, they promise each other never to tell. That evening during a dinner celebrating the store's successful opening, Michael's world explodes. His father is called and told that the store is burning out of control. As the family reacts, Michael runs to his grandfather's house to seek comfort. There Michael confesses. His grandfather summons his father and tells Michael he must now tell his father about what he has done. The world stands still as the boy haltingly faces his father. We are amazed by his courage.

As family therapists working with and writing about children, we are aware that we are privileged recorders and co-authors of children's stories. This is both an honor and a challenge in work that aspires to honor children's voices and knowledge. When a child or family consults us, we try to keep in mind the restraints of dominant cultural beliefs and theories about children and to look at the actions and stories we are told in the context of children's limited power.

Depending upon one's perspective, Michael's facing his father and taking responsibility for the fire is either an ordinary, taken-for-granted act of a child 'having' to tell a parent what he has done or an astonishing act of bravery.

From our perspective, children participate in acts of courage and trust daily, in families, at school, on playgrounds, and at childcare programs. These moments often go unnoticed in an adult-centered society. Since most children and their families enter therapy because of problems in their lives, we find it useful to bring events and family members' understanding of those events into a space to be questioned and reconsidered.

In this chapter we illustrate therapeutic work with children using narrative ideas. We discuss the collaboration with one child, Daniel, and his family. There are limitations in using a single example, since every situation is unique (a particular child, in a particular family, in a particular classroom, in a particular school, in a particular culture). However, the problems Daniel faces are familiar to most therapists seeing children and families. Through the interviews and examples of Daniel's developing a new lived narrative, we offer the reader a journey through this work. Our hope is that Daniel's story reflects the potency of narrative ideas and practices for creativity, collaboration, and celebration of children's strengths.

The narrative approach

Our work is based on social constructionist ideas (Berger & Luckmann 1966; Gergen 1985; Hoffman 1990) and narrative practices (Anderson & Goolishian 1988; Bruner 1991; Freedman & Combs 1996; Hoffman 1991; Monk, Winslade, & Crocket 1996; White 1995; White & Epston 1990; Zimmerman & Dickerson 1996). Social constructionist ideas include: (1) a person's sense of self is constructed through interaction with others; (2) realities are socially constructed; (3) realities are constituted through language; (4) there are no essential truths; and (5) realities are organized and maintained through narrative (Freedman & Combs 1996). We think of 'story' instead of pattern or labeling; of 'society' rather than system.

Any narrative is an act of bridging, connecting the teller, who in therapy is the person with intimate knowledge of the experience, and the listener, who is the therapist. The more narrative is studied, the more one realizes how very complex this bridging actually is, and how much our lives are shaped by such experiences, both for the teller and the listener. People come to therapy because of a problem that is bothersome and restraining to their life. The therapist tries to understand the influence of the restraints and provide an interaction with the teller where a co-construction of a preferred description can originate, take shape, and be acted upon.

As narrative therapists, we are concerned with meaning rather than generalizations or assumptions. We are interested in exceptions rather than similarities so we choose to look at specific contextualized details. We interview family members in the presence of each other (or about one another), seeking descriptions, beliefs, ideas, and perceptions of experiences. The perceptions of each person – therapist, interviewee, and listener – are relationally shaped by the presence of the others. It is more important to approach families with all of these ideas about therapy in mind, than to practice any particular narrative technique (Combs & Freedman 1998). The culture each one of us lives in plays a tremendous role as a transmitter of ideas, expectations and stories that people tend to experience as taken-for-granted realities.

As members of families, neighborhoods and religious institutions, children are not exempt from these influences of the social world. Additionally, they are constantly exposed to the media. Outside of their families, schools are often the primary institutions where children are saturated in cultural narratives and witness cultural practices for extended periods of time each day. We do not suggest that teachers or schools 'cause' problems for children, but we do think that exploration of school as part of a child's cultural context is fitting. For example, educators in Western cultures are socialized to see the formal curriculum as the core of what they do. While students may be attempting to study the curriculum, they are also engaged in life at school. Chris McLean (1995) points out how the educators' approach that considers underfed, poorly clothed, and inadequately supervised children as 'unteachable' hides the reality that, for working-class and poor children, school can represent a hostile, class-based structure of authority and privilege to which they have no access. Education in these schools literally requires these students to become 'class traitors'. While this dilemma is very different than the one we describe in this chapter, it is illustrative of the way the dominant culture can create a context for problematic life stories to evolve.

When working with children and their families, it is also important to think about how dominant discourses affect our work. To name a few: the role of adults in relation to children is 'instructional' (therefore interpretive and serious); children need to be 'socialized' (so approaches need to be methodical); children are not old or wise enough to 'know' things (so adults tell them what they should think or feel); and adult time is more 'precious'. If we as therapists get caught up in these assumptions we can unwittingly contribute to a child's experience of having little power in his or her own life.

Clearly we cannot change a child's culture in our office, but we can create a different kind of social interaction in which a child's knowledge is given greater value. We strive to stay mindful of our input and exercise responsibility regarding the weight of our influence in shaping children's lives and the narratives by which they describe their lives (Loptson & Stacey 1995).

Opening space for preferred stories

We are interested in helping people deconstruct the problematic stories they are experiencing and construct preferred stories. We use a number of practices to that end. We use questions to gain clarity of understanding and to offer linguistic options for expanding possible meanings (Stacey 1995). We also name problems and have externalizing conversations about them (Doan & Clifton 1990; Durrant 1989; Epston 1992; White 1989). That is, we invite family members to join us in seeing problems as separate from people and to use therapy as a context in which to renegotiate the relationship with the problem. In so doing, we are turning a dominant cultural practice on its head. Rather than seeing the child as a problem we are inviting the family to join with the child in standing up to the problem. This helps eliminate blame and defensiveness and frees a child for more personal agency (Tomm 1989). It helps family members unite with each other against problems instead of being torn apart by them or demonizing the child.

Once problems are exposed in this way, family members are free to recognize and construct preferred stories (Dickerson 1996). It is useful to create an audience for these alternative stories and work to commemorate and celebrate change.

As we describe the example of our work with Daniel, we intersperse commentary about these ideas with descriptions of the work.

Case illustration: Daniel's story

Daniel's mother, Evelyn, called Virginia to request therapy for Daniel after psychological testing and a series of school meetings. Evelyn explained that Daniel was having difficulty with academic requirements, as well as his behavior. Testing had revealed that Daniel had difficulty with verbal memory, verbal processing, and oral formulation skills. He had been engaged in speech and language intervention to learn techniques for enhancing processing of language and memory strategies. He was meeting with a resource teacher at school and had weekly tutoring after school. Evelyn expressed more concern about the anger and discouragement she saw in her son. Virginia arranged a meeting with Evelyn and Daniel. Daniel's father, Alex, traveled extensively as part of his work, and was unable to attend most of the therapy meetings.

At the time of the first meeting, Daniel was a nine-and-a-half-year-old boy who looked at least two years older. At first, he was cordial but not interested in talking, so initially the conversation was with Evelyn. She described her serious concern about the discouragement she saw in Daniel, the difficulty he was having in the classes, and the fights he was having at school. She said Daniel was 'being teased and fighting back'. He had gotten in trouble a number of times at school, most often on the playground or as school was letting out in the afternoon. However, the general discouragement about school had her deeply concerned. She began to experience helplessness and felt at a loss about what to do.

After Evelyn described her perceptions of the problem, Virginia hoped that Daniel might be ready to talk, so she began addressing questions to him.

We like to begin therapy by finding out about the life of family members separate from the problems that bring them to therapy. Hearing what they enjoy and are interested in helps all of us to avoid letting the problem color our ideas about family members. In this situation, Daniel declined to participate in this kind of conversation and Evelyn quickly began describing the problem. Rather than forcefully interrupt and redirect her, Virginia listened.

It is also our practice to ask children if there is a problem and how they would describe it. Virginia begins with the first of a cluster of problems described by the mother in order to understand Daniel's experience. In so doing, we acknowledge children as privileged authorities on their own experience. Thus, Virginia is interested in turning the conversation to Daniel as soon as he is willing to speak.

THERAPIST: Daniel, can I ask you some questions now? I remember you didn't want to talk when you first got here. I'm just not clear on some things, and would like to ask you. Would you talk now?

DANIEL: Yes, I guess so.

THERAPIST: How long has the problem of not understanding some things at school been giving you trouble?

DANIEL: A long time.

THERAPIST: Since kindergarten?

DANIEL: No, not *that* long.... I don't know.

THERAPIST: Since second grade? Do you remember second grade?

DANIEL: Yes, but it wasn't second grade.

THERAPIST: Not second grade either?

DANIEL: No, just before school was out last year.

THERAPIST: The end of third grade, then? *(At this point, Daniel is in the second month of fourth grade.)*

DANIEL: Yeah. *(Evelyn also nods yes.)*

THERAPIST: So tell me what happens. Is it just in certain classes?

DANIEL: Just sometimes, not all the time.

THERAPIST: So there are times you are free of the problems?

DANIEL: Yes.

THERAPIST: Really? Could I ask you some about this?

DANIEL: Yes.

THERAPIST: So Daniel, when are you free from them?

DANIEL: When I'm playing with my friends ... when I'm playing hockey, and with my mom or my dad.

Since the mother had described a cluster of problems Virginia began with the first one, and then, rather than naming a specific problem, she quickly initiated an externalizing conversation by calling it 'the problem' or 'the problems'.

THERAPIST: So you play hockey? What position do you play? Do you play on a team? *(They talk of hockey. Daniel loves hockey; he has been skating since an early age and has been playing team hockey since he was 7. Alex played hockey from childhood through college. Daniel talks about his favorite professional players. He and Evelyn educate Virginia, since she knows little about hockey.)*

The conversation about hockey helps to minimize the hierarchy inherent in therapy contexts (Cohen, Combs, DeLaurenti, DeLaurenti, Freedman, Larimer & Shulman 1998). It reminds everyone that there are subjects in which Daniel is an expert and Virginia is not. It also reminds Daniel of happy stories in his life, which will undoubtedly be useful in changing his relationship with the problem.

THERAPIST: Daniel, what happens when the problem comes?

DANIEL: It's in math. I just have to ask questions and I don't get to ... because by the time I try and see if I can do it and I can't I just get mad ... Then the teacher doesn't want me interrupting ... and then she says it's time to do something else. I *really* get mad then. *(Then he blurts out)* I just have low confidence.

THERAPIST: *(Thoughtfully)* What does that mean, low confidence?

DANIEL: When I just don't want to try anymore.

THERAPIST: Did you think of this or did someone tell you? I mean is that the word that tells how you're feeling just then?

DANIEL: Yeah, for *that,* yeah.

THERAPIST: What about the anger, what happens to the anger then?

DANIEL: I don't know – I just get mad, and then when people tease, I fight.

THERAPIST: The other kids tease? Do they tease you about the schoolwork?

DANIEL: Yes, and other things too.

EVELYN: I think it's because he is big, and the other boys test that.

THERAPIST: How does the anger work? Does the anger come along with low confidence?

DANIEL: *(Dropping his head and speaking in a quieter voice)* Yeah, like a secret mission against me.

THERAPIST: A secret mission? So do you know when it's coming?

DANIEL: No.

In the externalizing conversation two candidate names are used for the problem: 'anger' and 'low confidence'. As the work continues Daniel settles on 'temper' and 'low self-confidence'. Virginia is interested in mapping the effects of the temper and low self-confidence in Daniel's life.

Deconstructing the problem

In clarifying and writing down Daniel's words, Virginia thinks of her work as collaborating with Daniel in creating a document of his unique knowledge about the problems. It is this idea that becomes central in the document created. The 'Temper's Secret Mission with Low Self-Confidence' document was developed over a number of sessions, with Evelyn in a listening position or with only Daniel and Virginia present when he requested time alone. The conversations through which the document was developed were playful and included a sense of struggling with a mystery. It was clear to everyone involved that personifying the problem and thinking about the problem as having a secret mission was Daniel's inspiration. The therapist joined in, asking questions to help Daniel fill in and expand his ideas (Griffith & Griffith 1994). The document is written as if the problem is speaking. As Daniel examined the situation from the perspective of the problem, he gained ideas and descriptions of the mission that made the problem less confusing and overwhelming to him.

Temper's secret mission with low self-confidence against Daniel

The mission of temper and low self-confidence: *To hide and sneak around Daniel Green for an invasion at any shaky moment.*

1. At the slightest quiver in Daniel, we move in closer, putting thoughts in Daniel's mind. We have him doubt his abilities; we have him think others don't look up to him, honor him, or care that much. We talk him into thinking he can't do something,
2. The biggest trick we pull is keeping Daniel thinking these thoughts, so he won't think about what he needs at the time. This is called the fake-it method.
3. Because we are so klutzy, we have to be careful, so he won't notice. We usually send frustration and irritation first. If Daniel falls for those we know we have a better chance to get him. (This was documented after Daniel really began to catch onto the methods temper was using in its mission.)

4. We know when Daniel is not fully dedicated to the task. We can sense his weakest moments, when he feels the pressure of time or impatience creeping in. (This was documented after a setback.)

Through the process of creating this document, Daniel and Virginia deconstruct the problem (White & Epston 1992) by illuminating its construction (Brooks 1984). We assume that there are always counterplots or events that would not be predicted by problem-saturated stories. As the deconstruction was going on, Virginia was alert to any events or experiences that stood outside of the problem-saturated story.

A possible alternative story

Virginia was interested in the times and ways Daniel had escaped from temper and low self-confidence. When asked about times when temper and low self-confidence were not around, Evelyn spontaneously announced that temper was completely absent during hockey. Virginia explored this further, asking Daniel for details about how he dealt with temper during hockey. She discovered that Daniel had no problems with temper during hockey practice or games or when playing with friends at home. Virginia asked him what made the difference in those situations. They discovered that, although hockey was quite competitive, Daniel was confident and was enjoying the situation, and his favorite professional player never lost his temper.

Daniel also said his coach was a 'fair person'. This seemed important to Daniel, so Virginia asked about the meaning of this. Daniel meant not only that the coach followed a set of rules to determine consequences, but that he also had experienced the coach as having a fair and flexible way of addressing conflicts. Further comparative questions were then asked about his experience of school in order to understand what was troubling him about the situation. Although the playground was supposed to be a place to be with friends, forget academic struggles, and have fun, instead it had become a place where Daniel experienced fierce competition. Evelyn believed this was partly due to his size. Daniel told of three boys in his grade who regularly picked on other boys but rarely got into trouble because the playground monitor did not see them initiate it. More often the boy being taunted would get into trouble after defensively striking out. There was also the dilemma of a 'no telling' code. ('Tattletales' are sometimes scorned in elementary schools, not just by other children, but by adults as well.)

Nevertheless, Daniel had proved that it was possible to get the best of temper. He had been able to do it in hockey and at home. An examination of how he did it in these two contexts was instrumental in developing the following 'counter-document'.

Daniel's secret mission against temper and low self-confidence

Daniel knows to be watchful of the tentacles of temper and low self-confidence.

1. He says to himself, 'This is just one thing' over and over and believes it. He reminds himself that whatever it is, 'it won't kill you'. [This second sentence was a later addition.]
2. Daniel promises his mom and dad that he will hold their love and strength in his heart for tough moments. But more importantly, he remembers the promise to himself to hold love and strength in his heart and stay strongly committed to this for those times when he *really* has to fight temper and low self-confidence.
3. When someone trips him or teases him, Daniel asks, 'Why did you do that?' This lets the person know he noticed but will *not* react back. Or he may say, 'You had no reason to ...' Other times Daniel makes himself not hear. (This is an advanced skill that came after much practice.)
4. Daniel has learned he cannot say 'It won't work' and refuse to try with ALL his strength. He has to believe and say 'I've *really* got to try this'. Then when he believes, he starts feeling better. He reminds himself, 'Don't get lazy, I have to do this every day'.
5. Because temper is klutzy Daniel can sense when it is coming. He becomes irritated and frustrated, and he experiences more body movement, like jiggling and wiggling and he talks back. Then it's got him. Staying quiet helps Daniel deal with temper.

6. When kids are teasing, it's easy to get caught up in doing the same. Instead, he must not tease, because it comes back at him when he least expects it. The best thing to do is to stay quiet or stay away.
7. It is important to this mission to talk about what is making the jiggling and wiggling. He has to decide to speak with a caring person, either a trusted friend or concerned adult. Daniel cannot hide and must speak up, so others know.

Composing the counter-document seemed to help generate hope and mastery for Daniel. The therapist works with the child's interest. If at some point the interest tangibly fades for the child, the therapist makes accommodations accordingly. Several ideas may be tried before one seems to fit. If the document or idea seems no longer useful, it is abandoned for new developments. When asked about his interest in the ideas described by the mission statements. Daniel said it helped him understand what was happening.

Circulating the new story

Because Daniel's father, Alex, was not able to attend therapy sessions, some of the sessions were videotaped so that Alex could watch them. Daniel told Virginia that his dad was encouraging his secret mission project and had gone over the document with him. Daniel said this helped him know what he was up against and helped him know of his father's faith in him. Later in the therapy, Daniel talked about the significance of including his parents. He said that when his parents understood what he was up against and what he and they could do about it, they encouraged him rather than wondering what to do.

Although some models of family therapy believe a parent is uninvolved or resistant if he or she does not attend therapy sessions, we do not make that assumption. We also do not necessarily focus on family relationships or assume that they are part of the problem. We do assume that the more people involved in the preferred story the better. For that reason we are very interested in people witnessing and participating in the development of the preferred story. Evelyn did this by being in a listening and reflecting position in the sessions. Alex did this by watching videotapes and talking with Daniel about them.

Although Virginia met with the school staff, the meeting was focused on academics. Daniel's grades and study skills were improving, and it was determined that he would continue with the part-time resource person. She had also become someone he liked talking with.

The school social worker was identified as an alternate person for Daniel to talk with as needed (this fitted with point 7 in Daniel's secret mission). As Daniel experienced more positive changes in his life, he and his mom decided to share the secret mission document with the school social worker in an attempt to spread the news of his work. They thought this would help the project along at school. The social worker was supportive and had noticed positive changes in Daniel, but for unknown reasons she did not communicate with his teachers or principal.

Alternatives to the problem-saturated story: A step of bravery

Daniel had been free of difficulty for well over a month when a problem erupted at school and Evelyn was called in to see the principal. Apparently Daniel had been pushed while standing in the line in the hallway. No one knew how or why this happened. For Daniel it had come out of nowhere, although the other boy was known for having problems with temper. Daniel pushed the boy back, on the leg, as the other boy tried to kick him. The other child started yelling curses and pushing others as well. As the other boy was taken to the office by the teacher, the other kids began snickering and laughing. Although Daniel was not implicated, later, after the teacher returned, he asked to go down to the principal's office 'because he felt bad for the other boy being taunted' and to take 'responsibility for pushing back'. This is an interview about Daniel's stand against temper and low self-confidence, about Daniel's own mission being practiced in a wider, more noticeable way. The following transcript is part of the therapy session two days later:

EVELYN: He asked to go down there (the principal's office), even when he didn't have to. He could have just gotten out of it. The teacher, the social worker, everybody knows that now, too. I'm glad I was called. I was kind of worried that this would be interpreted like the times before.

THERAPIST: I could see how it could be worrisome. Did you feel like going down to the office was a pretty brave thing for Daniel to do?

EVELYN: Yes. *(Quietly)* I was very proud, too.

THERAPIST: It could have been passed over, just kind of dropped there. And you were proud?

EVELYN: I was very impressed. But you can see there is some kind of readjustment going on around recess again, a different person is out there and it reached that time, that point, where kids were at each other.

THERAPIST: Yes, but you know, Daniel, I'm wondering if all of these times when kids are teasing are also opportunities for anger and temper to squeeze back into your life big-time? You know, to try to take over again? And you haven't let it so far, is that right?

DANIEL: Yeah, I didn't.

THERAPIST: Would you say going down to talk, downstairs in the school office, was a brave thing to do? ... For you to try and reach out to somebody who was calling you names and curses?

DANIEL: Yeah, 'cause I know how it is ... what it feels like to be so mad ... Yep. It was.

THERAPIST: So Daniel, do you know how you are able to be brave like that?

DANIEL: I just say it, like ... I am part of it, because I did sort of push him back, on the leg. So I should go down to talk.

THERAPIST: Because you pushed him back, on the leg?

DANIEL: Yeah, I went down there. I was trying to help him feel better.

THERAPIST: So you went down and faced the adults who could have seen what you did as wrong?

DANIEL: *(Whispers)* I took responsibility.

THERAPIST: Yes, you did, and you also told the truth. You told them what you did, too.

DANIEL: Just to say ... I pushed him on the leg. The teachers said he had two weeks to be in (meaning two weeks of staying in from recess or after school) because he got so mad). He said I kicked him but I didn't.

THERAPIST: And you went down to explain?

DANIEL: Just to say that I pushed him back. I tried to tell him I understood, that it isn't how it ought to be, teasing and all ... but, he tried to kick me again when I was down there. In a way, he deserves it.

THERAPIST: Yeah, but Daniel, you know what I'm saying? Instead of letting him tell a big whopper (lie) and not say anything because you were not in trouble, for you to go down to the office and tell them the truth about your reaction and also offer understanding to him, was that a pretty brave thing to do?

DANIEL: Yeah.

THERAPIST: What do you think makes it brave?

DANIEL: That I decided to go down. Because, I mean, I didn't really have to.

THERAPIST: You could take half responsibility on it?

DANIEL: Or none at all.

THERAPIST; Right.

DANIEL: But I just thought I'd have part of it.

THERAPIST: So you were willing to take the responsibility in that way?

DANIEL: Yeah.

THERAPIST: *(To Evelyn)* You know, you talked about this last time. His directness. What was it you said? I can't remember the exact words, where you said Daniel ...

EVELYN: That he is very honest.

THERAPIST: Yes, and he didn't stay silent about this, that he said it outwardly at school. Earlier you said you really appreciated this about Daniel. That you felt good about his honesty and being able to trust him. It sounds like in this situation it was also a brave thing because it could have really backfired, right? Daniel, how did you stand your ground about this? How did you do it?

DANIEL: Well, when he said the 'F' and 'B' words, I just stood there.

Everyone was laughing. I didn't laugh or anything.

THERAPIST: Really?

DANIEL: Just stood there.

THERAPIST: Now, was that the not-hearing strategy you talked about (looking at the mission list)? You know where you stop hearing?

DANIEL: Yeah. It was.

THERAPIST: Wow. Good for you. So, Daniel is there some way we need to add this not-hearing strategy to this list of the things for your mission? You remember this list?

DANIEL: Yeah.

THERAPIST: What do we add to this, do you think? Do you want me to read what we have?

DANIEL: Yeah.

THERAPIST: Say to yourself 'this is just one thing' over and over again, until you believe it, You have to believe it.

DANIEL: And it won't kill you.

THERAPIST: Oh, and it won't kill you *(adding this to the first point in the mission document).*

THERAPIST: Was holding your parents' strength and love in your heart operating today, also?

DANIEL: I said, 'Forget it'. It just kind of came to me.

THERAPIST: Really? It just came from inside you?

DANIEL: Sure.

THERAPIST: So, do you think that's a good thing? That it just came from inside you?

DANIEL: Yeah. It was just there helping me with other people.

The story of this incident is an alternative to the problem-saturated story (de Shazer 1991; Morgan 1995). It speaks to Daniel's bravery (Radke-Yarrow, Zahn-Waxler, & Chapman 1983), whereas the problem-saturated story was about temper and low self-confidence. The transcript illustrates questions asked to facilitate the retelling of this preferred story in detail and making meaning from it.

Later in the session Virginia became aware that she had made an assumption from her own response to hearing the story. The collaboration of narrative work includes the therapist openly questioning and correcting his or her own motivations or assumptions. She had introduced the word bravery and wondered if it was fitting for Daniel. Daniel responded, '1 didn't go out and slay a dragon'. Virginia then asked Evelyn about her ideas regarding bravery. She spoke of regular people who had shown some compassion for others. Virginia wondered if another term might be better, rather than imposing the term 'bravery' on Daniel, but Daniel changed his mind, declaring, 'It does count as a *step* of bravery'.

As Dugan & Coles (1989), Freeman, Epston, and Lobovits (1997), Garbarino, Dubrow, Kostelny & Pardo (1992) and others warn us, we do not want to romanticize young people or make them into heroes. Virginia's aim is to be respectfully attentive and to appreciate what Daniel is doing and thinking, but not overstate it. We do admit, however, there are times when we are astonished at what children think and how they are able to quickly redirect themselves. It is especially during these moments with children that we realize we are privileged to be speaking with them about their rediscovered personal agency.

Interviewing the problem

Interviewing the problem is something that can be done at different points in the therapy. It can be done early on to expose the way the problem works or later to build motivation in the fight against the problem. Daniel had minor setbacks and then three weeks free of trouble. As a way of expanding Daniel's newfound freedom from the problem, Virginia asked if she could interview the problem. (Roth & Epston 1996a, 1996b; Zimmerman & Dickerson 1997). Pretending to be the problem offers the child a playful perspective about the experience of success.

In the following dialogue, Daniel is being interviewed alone; in the first part of the session Evelyn had told Virginia that the family would be moving and she wanted Daniel to have some time alone with her.

THERAPIST:. This is just an idea. What if you pretend you're the temper? Would you be temper and low self-confidence?

DANIEL: What do you mean?

THERAPIST: You let me interview you ... You be temper and low self-confidence and let me interview you.

DANIEL: Do what?

THERAPIST: You be temper. As temper you have had a secret mission against Daniel, right?

DANIEL: Oh ... yeah *(half smiling)*.

THERAPIST: Along with low self-confidence, you have had this mission, right? Against Daniel?

DANIEL: Sure *(with more enthusiasm)*.

THERAPIST: Okay, I'm going to be the interviewer. Temper, is Daniel right that you and low self-confidence decided to hide and sneak around him?

DANEL: Yes, but now I'm dying *(gasping and holding his throat)*.

THERAPIST: You're dying?

DANIEL: Yes *(slumping back in the chair)*.

THERAPIST: Are you croaking for real? Okay, you're taking some of your last breaths, are you? Well listen, before you draw your last breath, can you just tell me one thing? Daniel has struggled with you for a while and then not. Would you say that you really put up a good fight with him?

DANIEL: Ahh, yeah, yes I did *(draping across one arm of the chair)*.

THERAPIST: Did you or did you not try to take over his life?

DANIEL: Yeah, I did.

THERAPIST: And you're saying now he's won? Hmm, you're giving up?

DANIEL: Forfeiting *(raspy-voiced)*.

THERAPIST: You're forfeiting! So you are going to forfeit and walk off, have I got this right?

DANIEL: Uh-huh.

THERAPIST: Tell me *(trying to match some of his drama),* what strategy did Daniel use? I mean, what did he use to get you on the run? Was it some double moves? Or did he bring a lot of defensive action play against you? Or did he have some other kind of strategy to finally *get* you?

DANIEL: He ... he ... he had self-confidence.

THERAPIST: He had self-confidence, so he believed in himself. You decided that was enough for you! Temper, do you think you put up a good fight to get him? Do you think you've tried your lowest, sneakiest, and sleaziest ways with Daniel? Do you think you've practiced your most famous types of strategies against him?

DANIEL: *(Whispers)* This, this is the first time *(sigh)* I have *ever* lost.

THERAPIST: The first time you've ever lost! Unfortunate, uh-huh. Well, does it feel like some relief that you're going, that you're off, you're truly done?

DANIEL: Sort of *(whining)*.

THERAPIST: Some relief about that for you?

DANIEL: Yeah.

THERAPIST: Is Daniel a pretty tough match?

DANIEL: Yeah. I do like a round of torture.

THERAPIST: You do like a round of torture, huh? You're not coming back for another round are you? Have you tortured Daniel enough?

DANIEL: Yeah, 'cause I'm dying, 'cause I screwed up.

THERAPIST: So you made a mess of it? Did you make a mess of it, or did Daniel outsmart you?

DANIEL: Yeah, he outsmarted me.

THERAPIST; Yeah, he outsmarted you. Can we switch back now? Will you be Daniel now?

Interviewing the problem helped highlight and thicken the story of the defeat of the problem. Virginia followed the interview of the problem with questions about Daniel's experience of being temper and low self-confidence. He said that he enjoyed this experience and decided that temper probably doesn't die, but forfeits. He realized in reflecting about it that he needed to be ready because it could try to return during his upcoming move to a new house and new school. They talked further about his family moving.

Circulating the preferred story beyond the family

As Daniel and his family prepared for the move to a new community, one concern was Daniel's new school and the importance of the problems not following him there. In that regard, Evelyn was very upset when she saw that the current school had prepared a report to accompany Daniel to his new school. Except for a letter from the resource teacher, the six-page report focused on Daniel's academic deficits and on previous behavior problems. Both Evelyn and Virginia thought the report did not reflect Daniel's great progress. In therapy Daniel was recounting more and more examples of his handling difficult playground and after-school situations well. These triumphs seemed to be at odds with the report.

This disparity discouraged Evelyn and Alex. Evelyn believed that even if they explained their current perceptions of Daniel to the school, the report could contribute to a negative start for him. For Virginia, the disparity highlighted the imbalance of power between the well-intentioned institution meant to serve children and the child and family being served. As therapists we do not see ourselves as neutral, but rather as on the side of preferred stories. We also strive to be aware of our own power. In this situation, Virginia decided to redress the power imbalance between Daniel and the school. She did this by creating a letter that could be offered to the new school as an alternative report.

At the following session, when Virginia told Daniel about the letter, he was very interested in knowing what it said. Together, they read the initial draft, sentence by sentence. He asked what different words meant, such as 'socioemotional,' and 'inconsistent'. He wanted to know why the letter sounded so 'official'. Evelyn explained that it should be formal because they hoped it would become part of his record – what his new school principal and teachers would read about him. The purpose of this letter was to offer alternative examples of some of the things cited by the school report. The following is the text of the letter:

Re: Daniel Green
To whom it may concern:

I have worked with Daniel over the past six months regarding his socioemotional adjustments to increased academic demands and often unpredictable educational methods. The school environment was inconsistent in structuring teaching and learning situations that would allow Daniel to use his skills consistently. There had been recommendations by the psychologist of how to set the structure by giving instruction at both the auditory and visual levels with follow-up and progressive steps for learning. These were not translated to the classroom or special classes in computer lab or in long-term classroom assignments.

The difficulties Daniel originally experienced led him to feel overwhelmed and desperate. These feelings brought his self-confidence down, and he did not feel safe asking for help at the school for fear of being criticized and ostracized (both of which had occurred). In addition, the school had not provided predictable emotional support for him when these difficulties became apparent.

I have found Daniel to be an eager child who responds well when encouraged and given tools to solve situations. Daniel has many strengths. He is empathic toward others, he is a good negotiator and leader when structures allow it, and he is usually diligent in his work. If he thinks something is beyond him, anxiety can come to haunt him, but if given encouragement and ideas to work with, he can pursue solutions independently, with follow-up.

Even with the obstacles in his educational environment, Daniel has progressed academically according to grade-level standards in all subjects, with exceptional strength in math, writing, and social studies. He does have some challenges when writing lengthy assignments, where the organization of thoughts and ideas converge with tedious writing skills. Once in more advanced grades, he can use spell-check and other computer aids to check his work.

As an only child he is sensitive to issues of belonging in peer relationships. This is understandable, because he depends on these relationships more than children with siblings or physically close kinship networks do. He tolerates competition well when he is confident in what he is attempting, but can become disappointed in himself when there is less self-confidence about what he is doing or no clear understanding of the task.

Daniel has made incredible advances over the last several months, and has perceptions beyond his age about emotional and moral issues, such as injustice, prejudice, acceptance of differences, honor, and honesty. He has had a number of pressures at home, including moving to a new place, the death of an uncle he was close to, and the absence of his father over the last three months. Given these stresses, he has accomplished incredible control of his anxiety, frustration, and fears. Daniel has a brave spirit and fortitude, It has been a great pleasure knowing him.
Sincerely,
Virginia Simons, M.S.W.

After hearing the letter, Daniel leaned back in his chair and took a deep breath. He said he liked the letter and did not want to change any of it. Evelyn smiled and said that now she felt more prepared for discussions in the new school situation. She was happy that the new school staff would learn of Daniel's efforts before he arrived. For the two of them, having an alternative letter in 'official' language that could be read and re-read meant that the preferred version of Daniel's story could be circulated. Daniel would carry other convictions about himself to the new school within his heart and mind.

This is an example of a letter that thickens a preferred story and circulates it beyond the family. Most often we write therapeutic letters (Freeman, Epston, & Lobovits 1997; White & Epston 1990) directly to the person or family we are seeing in therapy. This letter, instead, shifts the news to a more public arena, where documents about Daniel are on file. Daniel's knowledge and acceptance of this letter is also a significant therapeutic step because he had been rather private about his efforts until now. The letter signals his willingness to go public. Virginia hoped that this would lead the way for a community of acknowledgment in his new school.

Consulting the consultant

As the work was drawing to an end, Virginia interviewed Daniel and Evelyn about therapy. This reinforced Daniel's status as an expert on his own experience in therapy (White & Epston 1992). Along with his consultation about the therapy experience, Daniel agreed to be a reference for others who might come in with similar problems (Epston 1992, pp.11-25). The following transcript is the section of the interview with Daniel.

THERAPIST: So, Daniel, would you tell me what it was like to come to counseling and being here, meeting and talking about all this?

DANIEL: Hell *(starts laughing, glancing over at his mom).*

EVELYN: *(Laughter)* 'Hell?!' *(To Virginia)* And you've got the camera rolling?

THERAPIST: I've got the camera rolling. *(Laughter; Daniel grins.)*

THERAPIST: So, Daniel, it was pretty hard, huh? What about it was hard?

DANIEL: It was hell the way I felt talking about the problem, figuring it out.

THERAPIST: Yeah, talking about the problem and what it was doing? What about the figuring it out? The mission? Daniel, if a kid were having difficulty would you advise him to come talk to somebody or not?

DANIEL: If they were having a problem everyday, yeah. If their parents don't know how to help, yes!

THERAPIST: So, if parents can't deal with it or can't seem to figure it out?

DANIEL: Yeah.

THERAPIST: Okay. So even though it was hard to talk, was it a good thing?

DANIEL: Oh, yeah. Tell them, once you start to know what is happening, it gets a little easier to come.

Reflecting on what happens in their world and facing and overcoming overwhelming odds may very well be hell for some children. Daniel's spontaneous summation of the experience holds wisdom for us all. Entering therapy can make children as well as adults feel at risk and vulnerable. When parents are present, perhaps it feels even more risky for children, who are in a less powerful position than adult clients.

Being in the role of consultant begins to redress the imbalance of power. This consultation acknowledges that the child has expertise about the experience. Daniel's interview thickened the narrative of him as a competent person (Seligman, Revick, Jaycox, & Gillham 1995). It was not done as a strategy or technique, but rather as a way to recognize the wisdom he possesses about himself.

Rituals and ceremonies

First introduced in narrative work by Michael White and David Epston (1990), celebrations and award- and prize-givings signal a shift of therapy's focus from the problematic relationships to the positive steps taken. This leads to future growth. The degree of focus on problems, and taking steps against them, compared to that on the preferred, alternative stories will vary according to the situation and motivations of the particular child and family. Marking out and highlighting accomplishments can be done through symbols.

As therapy was ending, Virginia mentioned the possibility of an award to honor his success (Freedman & Combs 1996; Freeman, Epston, & Lobovits 1997; White & Epston 1992), Being a hockey fan, Daniel immediately began talking about the Stanley Cup. In the following transcript of the final session, Virginia followed up on the idea.

THERAPIST: We talked a little bit about this Stanley Cup idea last time. Do you think we can figure out how to do this? The Stanley Cup is *big*. We can create one, but it would have to be smaller.

DANIEL: Sure.

THERAPIST: Like a little Stanley Cup award?

DANIEL: Yes, out of candy!

THERAPIST: Oh, a candy one? What kind of candy?

DANIEL: Chocolate.

EVELYN: Chocolate is his favorite.

THERAPIST: A chocolate Stanley Cup?

DANIEL: Yeah.

THERAPIST: Or something like that? Do you think it will be able to travel from here to your new house without melting? I'm thinking about that since you didn't want to get it until you are in school there, remember, so you know you have won, even in a new place. You said in two weeks?

DANIEL: I'll probably still be shy; wait more.

THERAPIST: Do you think we should wait longer than that? That you may still not be completely comfortable there?

DANIEL: Try three.

THERAPIST: Well, do you think anxiety could give temper a chance for a surprise visit?

DANIEL: Maybe.

EVELYN: We leave in a week, then settle in the new house, so it will be two weeks after starting at the new school.

THERAPIST: About three weeks then? We'll try for it to arrive after the beginning of going to the new school.

DANIEL: Maybe I could get it after the first week or two.

THERAPIST; Yes, if the post office cooperates.

EVELYN: Before you know the other kids that well.

DANIEL: Yeah, yeah.

THERAPIST: Okay. I'll try.

After the conversation about the Stanley Cup, Virginia presented Daniel with a copy of his certificate, since he preferred the original to be mailed with the Stanley Cup. To mark this time as a celebration, Virginia brought in a couple of balloons and a snack.

EVELYN: Wow *(responding to the balloons, soda, and a little package of 'Tikes' pencils).*

DANIEL: Yes-s-s *(spontaneously raising his arms and clasping his hands in a victory motion over each shoulder).*

(Virginia and Evelyn applaud.)

This ended the sessions with Daniel. The day before the family moved, Evelyn left a message indicating that Daniel had been talking with her about his experience and thoughts about moving. His leave-taking at school and with friends had been sad. Evelyn said she was sometimes amazed by his insights. He had been helpful to her as she dealt with her own emotions.

Virginia checked nearby shops but was unable to find a cup made of chocolate. Instead she sent Daniel a small trophy cup filled with chocolates and

Certificate of Bravery

This is to certify that

Daniel Green

has practiced numerous acts of personal bravery
in his fight for true, personal confidence in himself,
and that his story can be used
to give other children ideas about being brave.

Brave Persons Association of America

Dated this __________ day of________________, 20______

Signed: *Virginia A. Simons*

Virginia A. Simons, Sponsor

engraved, 'Stanley Cup of Bravery, Daniel'.[3] She enclosed the original bravery certificate in the box.

In a letter that Evelyn sent after the box arrived, she wrote that the trophy sits among Daniel's hockey trophies and other treasures on his shelf, where he chose for it to be. Daniel was surprised and delighted to find it filled with chocolate. Evelyn saved the certificate for his memory book.

About six months later Virginia wrote to Daniel to ask if she could talk about his experience with a group of therapists who were meeting to discuss ways to help children. Evelyn wrote back giving permission. The main thing Daniel wanted therapists and other adults to know is how bad bullying and teasing is for kids. 'It should not ever be allowed', Evelyn wrote. 'It is not allowed in his new school, and he thinks that made a big difference for him. All kids want things to be good, because if they are not you're hurt and unhappy. Oh, and hockey is still terrific.'

One year later, Evelyn wrote to say that after much soul-searching they were moving again to be near family. Both she and her husband had new jobs in the new community. Daniel had been on the B+ honor role for two grading periods and had been happy and doing well.

Conclusion

Using narrative ideas with children and families has repeatedly demonstrated that if we help people define problems, their experience can be the guide in authoring stories that stand outside the limits of those problems. Constructing preferred stories almost always goes hand in hand with the process of deconstruction. Once Daniel began to speculate and analyze the problem as external to himself, he could see places in life where he was already free of it. Acknowledging and concentrating upon these experiences that are exceptions to the problem can bring clarity, purpose, and direction to the therapeutic dialogues about the next steps to be taken. For Daniel this took the form of documents that both reveal the methods of the problem and declare his self-knowledge. The rest of the therapy included several narrative practices that allowed his story to be enriched, re-experienced, and shared.

Our hope in writing this chapter was to present a child's voice; Daniel's voice and his thinking, knowledge, and authorship of a preferred life story. Participating in Daniel's developments has made us aware that bravery does not have to speak in a loud voice or come from visibly grand demonstrations. His voice is one of many that reveal the abilities and knowledge accessible to us in children.

Notes

1. This chapter was originally published in *Children in Therapy: Using the family as a resource.* C. Everett Bailey, Ph.D., Editor, W.W. Norton & Company, New York, London, 2000.
2. Virginia A. Simons, M.S.W., is Clinical Instructor, Case Western Reserve University, Family Medicine Department, Fairview Center for Family Medicine, Cleveland, Ohio.
3. The total cost of this award, including postage, was less than $20.00, leading us to speculate on the benefits of including room for such expenditures in our practice budgets.

7

Lists[1]

This short paper describes some of the ways in which making lists within the therapeutic context has been helpful in our work with young children.

We were visiting with some friends and asked Sarah and Eli to tell us about their trip to the zoo that morning. 'We saw monkeys and giraffes and snakes', Eli said. 'Yeah, monkeys and alligators and a zebra', amended Sarah. 'And we ate hot dogs and Cokes and popsicles and popcorn',

Lists seem to be a natural way of keeping track of experience, especially for young people. When we first began to use narrative ideas (Combs & Freedman 1994; Dickerson & Zimmerman 1993; Epston 1989; Freedman & Combs 1996; Laird 1989; White 1995; White & Epston 1990; Zimmerman & Dickerson 1996) in working with children (Freeman, Epston, & Lobovits 1997; White 1984), our tendency was to take a list such as Eli's or Sarah's and ask questions to develop it into a storybook-like narrative of their trip to the zoo. While some children are astonishing in their memory of detail and can spontaneously provide rich narrative accounts, many others seem to prefer to recount their experience in the more condensed and efficient manner that lists make possible. Lists are a great way of working with these children's experiential worlds.

A list of accomplishments can bring forth vivid and meaningful experience of those accomplishments. In making a list with a child, the therapist helps to identify and name things that are worth listing. The process of writing these things down and reading them back makes them more 'real' and more memorable. Once written down, a list becomes a document (White & Epston 1990) that can be displayed, consulted, and circulated. A child can read a list and re-experience the knowledge it contains. She or he can see how big it is and count the number of items on it. If a list is worked on over the course of therapy, the child can see it grow. (See Freedman & Combs 1996, pp.232-236.)

We offer the following story to illustrate several ways in which lists may be brought forth and used. We have used this story previously (Freedman & Combs 1996) to illustrate other ideas.

Erica: A therapy story

Although the school had indicated that 9-year-old Erica[2] should be seen weekly by the school social worker, his caseload and Erica's class projects seemed to get in the way all too often. Grant and Diana, Erica's grandparents, worried that Erica might be 'depressed'. They decided to take matters into their own hands and brought Erica to see me (JF).

In a phone conversation before the first meeting, Ron, Erica's father, told me that he thought Erica needed something because she-seemed to 'always be cowering and not speak up', and her grades had plummeted. However, he and Erica's mother, Clarisse, and Erica's younger sister, Hannah, could not regularly attend our meetings because the couple worked different shifts, they were already in couple therapy, and Ron was in individual therapy and night school. The family had tried family therapy once and believed that it didn't work. Ron said that it was okay with them if Erica came to see me with his parents. We agreed to stay in touch by phone, and Ron indicated that the family would consider coming to occasional meetings.

The first meeting

At the first meeting, I began by asking Erica what she liked to do. She mumbled, 'I don't know', but did not disagree with her grandparents' list, which included art, drawing, singing, working on the computer, ice-skating, swimming, and rollerblading. Erica did volunteer that she didn't like her 7-year-old sister, Hannah. She didn't know if there was a problem, but listened quietly as Grant said, 'She doesn't give herself credit for anything. She never brags. She's always saying she's sorry – for nothing.' Diane added, 'She's very quiet. Hannah tells all of Erica's good news. Erica has nothing of her own because Hannah is always in on it.'

I asked Erica what she thought about what her grandparents said. She said she didn't know. When I asked several more questions, she finally said that she guessed she didn't give herself credit. I asked if she would be interested in making a picture to show what she didn't give herself credit for. She quietly drew on a large piece of newsprint a framed picture to represent her art, a report card, a bell to represent the bell chorus she was part of, a Taekwondo uniform because she was taking Taekwondo, a math book, and six friends.

I asked her about each of the elements of the drawing. She reluctantly told me that her grades in math were pretty good. Her grandparents agreed. She said that she didn't know whether the six kids she drew really were her friends or not, but in answer to questions she decided it was better to think they were because that would make her 'act on the other side', acting friendly instead of shy.

Erica did not seem interested in conversation about what kept her from taking credit for these things, so I asked her, 'If you could wave a magic wand that would help you start taking credit, what do you think you would notice that you are not noticing now?'

Erica quickly answered, 'I would be thinking on the happy side'. She explained that she would be seeing brighter colors, like a rainbow. She added a rainbow to the picture.

With further questioning she said that she'd feel better about going to Taekwondo and would be saying to herself, 'I'll do better than usual. I'll get my pattern right.'

Erica seemed to know so much about this that I asked her if the words she would say to herself were familiar ones. It turned out that just a few days before, she did a whole song in bell chorus without messing up once! She had said to herself, 'I'm going to do good', and she did. She thought that saying to herself, 'I'm going to do good', helped set the mood that would make her chances for 'doing good' great!

Erica's grandparents were delighted to hear that Erica already had taken a step toward giving herself credit. They knew she could do it, because she had in the past. To back this up, they recounted some experiences that they were delighted to hear about when Erica told about them in past years.

As they were getting ready to leave, I asked Erica if she wanted to take the picture home to remind her of what we had talked about. 'No, I want you to keep it', she said, looking down. 'But could I borrow the magic wand?' On my desk, she had spied my telephone companion, a clear tube full of glittering confetti suspended in a thick substance. I gave it to her.

The second meeting

At the second meeting, Erica was much more talkative. She told me that immediately after our first meeting she had forgotten about our conversation, but when she saw the magic wand she remembered. Then she reminded herself to take credit. The forgetting and remembering happened a few more times, and then she decided to carry the wand with her. She found out that '... it could make life better to give yourself credit. Then you won't always be mad at yourself.'
In the course of our conversation, we began calling the problem 'self-blame'. Erica saw that she was getting the best of the self-blame already. We developed the following list of ways that giving herself credit was making a difference in her life:

- It made it possible for her to keep doing what she already could do.
- It made her feel good about what she could do, rather than not letting it make any difference.
- It made her happy.
- It let her see that she was really good at Taekwondo.
- It helped her do a biography of her grandfather.

- It made her teachers notice and comment on how she was working harder.
- Maybe (she wasn't as sure about this one) it let her parents notice that she was doing better, because she had been feeling happier at home.

Grant and Diane added the following item to Erica's list:

- It helped her smile and talk to other kids, rather than stand quietly by herself when they picked her up from school.

We all wondered about where this project would make itself known next. Erica thought it might be with her sister. She told me, 'I might not always fight with her. I might stop getting mad at her for stuff she doesn't do.'

'So do you think the self-blame turns into blame against others sometimes?'

She nodded.

'And it gets you in fights too, huh?'

She nodded again.

'Wow. I didn't know it was so stressful. And you've already turned it around this much?'

Again she nodded.

'Do you think as you turn this blame around even more, you'll be more in touch with loving your sister?'

Erica nodded.

'Then what will happen?' I asked.

'Well', she confided, 'probably my parents will stop telling me I'll get coal in my stocking'. (It was December.)

I wondered if maybe the blame was messing up Hannah's life too. Diane and Grant thought maybe it was. We all agreed that it would be good for the whole family to know about how Erica was turning self-blame around and feeling better about herself. We agreed I would phone Ron and Clarisse and invite them and Hannah to the next meeting. We agreed that we would show them Erica's picture and fill them in on her 'feeling better about yourself' project.

The third meeting

Erica, Hannah, Clarisse, and Ron attended the third meeting. I had exacted Diane and Grant to come as well, but the family worked it out for just the four to come.

After I got to know Hannah, Clarisse, and Ron a bit, we unveiled Erica's pictorial list. Together, Erica and I described what the different images meant, and went over the list of what she had accomplished in regard to feeling better about herself.

Ron had already noticed a big difference in Erica. 'Erica has always tried hard', he said. 'But now she seems to be taking big steps'. He noticed that she had become more involved with kids her own age, whereas before she always seemed to be alone or with younger kids. He noticed her interacting more at the bell choir practice and Taekwondo. She began having guests over for the first time. Both he and Clarisse were happy about these developments.

I asked Ron what he thought this said about his daughter. He answered, 'She's becoming more mature'. He then added that she was also standing up for herself. He noticed her standing up for herself both with other kids and with Hannah.

Clarisse agreed in part, but said that she still hoped that the fighting, arguing, bickering, and whining between Erica and Hannah would stop.

I turned to Hannah and told her that Erica and I had had a conversation about how Erica thought that blame had come between them. She agreed. I wondered what effect the blame had on their sisterhood and whether this was something they might work on together. Erica blurted out, 'I don't want her coming. This is for me'. 'Would it be okay if you fill Hannah in on what we talk about that has to do with her, and the two of you see how you could work together?' I asked.

Erica nodded.

The fourth meeting

At the fourth meeting with Erica, Grant, and Diane, Erica updated me on areas she was feeling better about herself in. She added these items to her list:

- She got promoted to a green belt in Taekwondo.
- She got an 89 on a report she had done.
- She felt happy most of the time!

As there was now more that she was taking credit for, she updated her picture. She added a stage for being in a play, a snowflake for sledding, and 'NUBS is the best and so am I!' (NUBS was the name of a group she belonged to at her church.)

I asked a number of questions to fill out the story of how all of these changes were happening, what steps Erica was taking, what the turning points were, and how she was advising herself.

Erica shrugged in response. 'I still carry the magic wand. I remember the picture, and I look at my list.'

'What do they mean to you?' I asked.

'That I can do it', she said. 'That I can turn self-blame around.'

Again my attempts at co-authoring detailed narratives with Erica fell flat. Yet it was clear that she was progressing rapidly and that the therapy was helpful to her. I stopped asking re-authoring questions and invited her to develop some more lists.

I asked her if she would like to show me how much ground self-blame had before and how much it had now. I said, 'First, you could draw a box that would hold all the self-blame from before'.

She drew an oblong box.

'And what would be in it?' I asked.

Erica made this list inside tin box:

> Getting bad grades.
> Pictures aren't good.
> Fighting with sister.
> My parents fighting.
> Because I don't have any friends.

'So those are all the things that self-blame blamed you for?'

'Yes', said Erica, writing 'Before' in the box.

'How big of a box would it take to hold the self-blame in your life now?'

Erica drew a much smaller box.

'What's in it?' I asked.

'Fighting with my sister', she answered, filling the words in and adding 'Now'. She then drew a line through 'Getting bad grades', 'Pictures aren't good', 'My parents fighting', and 'Because I don't have any friends' in the first box, leaving only 'Fighting with sister'.

I showed the representation to Grant and Diane. 'Did you know Erica had shrunk self-blame this small?'

They had wondered but hadn't known for sure. We all speculated about the relative sizes of the two. The change had happened over the course of 9 weeks, so we wondered how long it would take to shrink the 'now' box, or if it was okay to leave it the size it was.

The fifth meeting

The fifth meeting took place 3 weeks later. In a phone call with Clarisse before this meeting, I discovered that Erica and Hannah were getting along much better and that Grant and Diane were on vacation. Clarisse volunteered to bring Erica to the meeting. I assumed we would meet together, but Clarisse dropped off Erica, so I saw her alone.

Erica told me that the most important thing that happened since the fourth meeting was that she made a lot of new friends. At this point in the therapy, I was quite aware of Erica's preferred style of communication. Rather than attempting to draw her out about an experience with a friend or asking questions about how she was going about making friends, I joined her in making this list of new friends:

Alison	Heather	Demetria
Emily	Vera	Antonio
Ilana	Stephanie	Reed
Brooke	Hannah	Sam
Enid	Melissa	Matt
Natalie	Dawn	Aaron
Shannon	Yukiko	Hayden
Morgan	Christina	Frank
Mara	Ginger	Robert
Sean		

Once the list of friends was documented, I asked Erica a few questions to fill in some detail. I learned that Erica was able to make all of these friends just by being herself. What she learned was 'Don't act like you're somebody else'. The self-blame got her to try to act like somebody else. The work she began in therapy helped her be herself.

We made a list of the main differences between this year and the last for Erica:

- Now she felt better about herself.
- She appreciated herself more.
- She had better grades.
- She had more friends.

She said that her parents and teachers noticed and that her grandparents would notice when they came back from vacation.

When I turned the conversation toward the relationship with Hannah, Erica said, 'But I told you. Now she's one of my friends'. I hadn't realized when she listed 'Hannah' that she was talking about her sister. Erica was very matter-of-fact about the old news that blame no longer was coming between her and her sister.

She thought that our work together was finished. We decided to meet one more time with the whole family to celebrate. I felt confident in making this suggestion, because of my previous conversation with Clarisse, who had confirmed that Erica was doing great.

The sixth meeting

At the sixth meeting, I announced that we were there to celebrate Erica's turning around self-blame and achieving the project of feeling better about herself! Erica showed the picture list again, describing it and pointing out the additions. She then read the list of accomplishments and the list of her friends' names. Hannah beamed when her name was read. After the reading was completed, Hannah confirmed that blame was gone from their relationship. She thought that Erica was mostly responsible, because she had been 'nicer and happier'. Everyone agreed this would make a big difference in family life.

Ron added that at the time the therapy began, the school was very concerned about Erica's performance. There had been talk of her possibly repeating the year. This prospect had been extremely distressing to Ron. He and Clarisse had contacted a Catholic school about the possibility of Erica's going there. They hoped that this would forestall her repeating a grade and that in a more structured program she would catch up. The Catholic school was not willing to admit Erica at grade level unless reports improved. Ron was relieved that at a parent-teacher conference just 2 days before, Erica's progress was characterized as excellent. He wondered if the therapy was responsible.

I said that we hadn't talked about school problems. I had known that Erica's grades were lower than in previous years, but I hadn't known the extent of this. I had spoken to the school social worker twice, but he had not mentioned academic problems. I said that it sounded to me like Erica was responsible for turning this around all by herself! She beamed.

We all had cookies that Diane supplied, and we congratulated Erica.

As the family was getting ready to leave, Erica handed me back my 'wand'.

'You can keep that', I said.

'I don't need it any more', Erica told me. 'The magic is here now', she said, patting her heart.

This therapy illustrates the use of a number of lists – the 'picture list', the list of ways in which giving herself credit was making a difference in Erica's life, the lists in the 'then' and 'now' boxes, the list of friends, and the list of differences between this year and last year. In the therapy with Erica, the lists were read and re-read. They were shared with other people, and she reviewed some of them between meetings. They served as concrete representations of portions of the work that seemed to make it more real and graspable.

An exercise

We offer the following exercise as a way of directly experiencing the usefulness of lists – even for adults. We hope that if you take the time to do this exercise and to become experientially involved in it, you will have some ideas about how you might use lists in working narratively with children.

This exercise will probably work best if you do it with another person, allowing her/him to guide you through it, talking with each other about your experience as you go. You can then switch roles and assume the guide/witness role for your partner. However, since you are probably reading this piece to yourself, we have written our suggestions as if you were doing the exercise by yourself.

Step I. Begin by identifying a problematic situation in your current life – a set of circumstances in which you experience yourself as stuck, unduly restrained, or not quite measuring up. Then set this situation aside for a few minutes. We will return to it later in the exercise.

Step 2. Remember what your life was like 5 years ago. Can you recollect what was going on in your life back then? Where were you living? What projects were you involved in? What were the important personal relationships in your life? What problems were you struggling with? (It is not important that you answer all these questions, or any of these specific questions. What is important for this exercise is that you remember your circumstances 5 years ago clearly enough to contrast them with your present circumstances.)

Step 3. Reflect for a few minutes on some of your experiences in moving from your circumstances of 5 years ago to those of today. We would guess that certain experiences stand out as memorable or important. For example, what do you know how to do that you didn't know how to do 5 years ago? What places are you familiar with that you weren't 5 years ago? Who do you know that you didn't know then? What have you accomplished? List these as they come to mind. As you look at the first few experiences on your list, do others come to mind? Add these to your list. What knowledge or skills did you learn in each experience on your list?

Step 4. Hang on to your list while you remind yourself of the situation from your present life that you identified in Step 1.

Step 5. If you really acknowledge and take ownership of the living knowledge that your list represents, what difference does that make in your experience of the problematic situation? What new possibilities do you see for how you will deal with that situation in the future?

Step 6. Reflect on the exercise and the helpfulness of using lists. In both our therapy story and our exercise, we have hoped to illustrate the usefulness of lists in documenting 'story-worthy' experiences. Do you think you will keep lists on your list of ways to work in doing therapy with children?

Editorial questions

Q: *(CS) Among the things that jumped out at me in this chapter and that impress me about your work in general are your flexibility and creativity! For instance, throughout earlier sessions you co-constructed Erica's externalized 'self- blame'. In response to your question of what her next step might be with this 'self-blame', she threw a new twist in by saying that her next step was wanting not to get as angry with her sister. But you were adept enough at this transition to ask her if her 'self-blame' sometimes turned into 'blame against others'. In another similar instance, Erica had understandable worry that her sister might assume too large a presence in her therapy. She suddenly declared that she didn't want her sister coming to therapy any more. Rather than become adamant that she come or completely dismissing her sister's participation altogether, you respectfully asked whether it was okay if Erica told her sister only what pertained to her sister and their relationship together.*

Another example of your creativity is your emphasis on list making with children. From my reading, it appeared that you chose this emphasis with Erica as a way to honor her matter-of-fact communication style with you. Is this so? You contrast list-making questions with 'co-authoring detailed narratives', which could involve such things as asking 'meaning questions' (Freedman & Combs 1996, pp.136-139) about her personal characteristics or values enabling her to do the things on her list. As you think about your work with children currently, how might you go about deciding whether to focus more on different verbal and pictorial list-making questions, and when to attempt to thicken clients' stories by asking 'meaning' and other questions? Do these two emphases (list-making and story-developing questions) overlap at times?

A: Thank you for your appreciation of our work. I (JF) did choose list making because it matched Erica's style. We hope that our decisions to ask questions or invite children to make lists or other symbolic representations follow from their styles. We move into particular ways of working simply by trying one way and moving to another if the first doesn't work. We are both 'talkers', so we usually start by inviting people to talk with us. If we notice that a child responds in lists, we will probably start thinking in terms of lists. If he or she tells stories, we will think more in terms of story development and meaning questions. If a child gives very brief answers to our questions or seems uncomfortable talking very expansively, we will usually think more about lists or using symbols (see Freedman & Combs 1996, pp.224-236). We do find that sometimes when we have developed more of a relationship with particular children, they talk more and in more detail. Then we might move from making lists to asking more story development and meaning questions.

Q: *(CS) One frequent thing that supervisees ask is how to respond when children give a host of 'I don't knows', shrugs, or all-too-brief answers to all our efforts! I noticed you did a variety of things in Erica's therapy at these times. You turned to her grandparents in the session and asked them to provide examples of things she liked to do, which 'helped join with her as a human being rather than as a 'patient'. You sidestepped verbalization by inviting her to draw the territory of 'self-blame' in the past and currently, and then to make a written list of what was in these boxes. You also asked a hypothetical, future-oriented question at one point.*

Can you share what sorts of things you think about when a child is reluctant to talk in therapy? Are there other things you have done at these times as well? Is there any pattern or similarity in the things you might attempt to do at these times? How important do you think it is to try to involve family and other 'audience' members when children are more reserved or in general? If this is significant for you, can you share a couple of ways you might go about this?

A: Perhaps the most important things we think about when a child is reluctant to talk in therapy are the prevalence and power of discourses that work to rob children of their voices: the 'Children should be seen and not heard' discourse, the 'Father knows best' discourse, the 'Children's knowledge is primitive knowledge' discourse, the 'Good students sit still, don't talk, and obey all the rules' discourse, and others. These discourses are insidious, and can very easily overwhelm our belief that children have lots of knowledge that is worth listening to.

It is a rare child who hasn't been silenced to some degree by these discourses, so it is no surprise at all to us when children are reluctant to talk – we expect this to be the case, especially in the beginning of therapy. However, we don't believe that this means that children have nothing worthwhile to say, or that they will *remain* reluctant to talk. Usually a child just needs a little proof that we are really interested in what he/she has to say.

Our earlier work was using Ericksonian therapy, and Milton Erickson believed that whatever the person said or did was a 'perfect' response. That early training was helpful in keeping us from feeling rejected or hopeless when someone doesn't show much verbal response. When a child is reluctant to talk in therapy, we wonder both how and what she/he is communicating and how we can adjust our communication style to be more compatible with hers/his. One of the things we might do in addition to introducing lists is to offer some possibilities ourselves and ask the child if we are right, or to choose from a number of possibilities. We do think audience is important for all of us, and particularly for children. One way I (JF) included the family with an 11-year-old who wanted to be seen alone was at the end of therapy to make a tape reflecting back on our work, which the child then shared with her family.

Q: *(CS) I know that a lot of your work with adults involves respectfully opening space for them to consider whether various sociocultural ways of being are currently useful in their lives. Erica was initially described as struggling with self-blame and not feeling entitled to much of a voice. If Erica had been 16 instead of 9 years old, do you think you might have tried asking her about whether she perceived her struggles as related to larger gender issues? If so, how might you have tried to do this?*

If she didn't find these questions helpful and gave matter-of-fact replies once more, might you have let the more overt sociocultural questions go for now and returned to your list-making questions or other sorts of questions, or might you have persisted with the former questions? What sorts of indicators might you use to determine whether you want to pursue sociocultural issues with children and adolescents (e.g., age, maturity, etc.)? In this or other situations, could you envision yourselves combining these sociocultural and list-making questions?

A: Before we answer any of these questions, we want to respond to your presupposition that the way we address sociocultural issues in therapy is directly, by asking questions that attempt to tie people's particular problems to general social issues such as gender inequality. Although we sometimes do this, we are more concerned that we be *thinking about* limiting or oppressive discourses as we sit with people.

We believe that it is our responsibility to be aware of as many of the potentially problematic discourses that affect people as we can, and to facilitate life narratives that are relatively unencumbered by such discourses. (See Hare-Mustin 1994 for an excellent discussion of this.) For example, we are aware of at least two commonly encountered discourses that might have been depriving Erica of her voice – the 'Adults know and children don't' discourse that we discussed in responding to your second set of questions, and those gender-based discourses that you refer to in this set of questions. The main way that we challenged these discourses with Erica was by not letting them make us deaf to her knowledge.

We didn't try to get her to link self-blame and voicelessness to either of these discourses; we used our knowledge of them to help us avoid their tricks. To the degree that we were able to avoid being tricked by them, we were able to believe that Erica had a voice and to find ways to help her use it. This would have been our basic stance, whether Erica was 9, 16, 32, or 64.

If she had been 16, we *might* have invited her to examine self-blame and voicelessness in the light of her experience of patriarchy, and she might have found this useful, but what was of most importance to us about sociocultural issues would still have been whether or not *we* were aware of them and striving to keep them from closing down possibilities for how Erica might live her life. If we did decide to ask her whether she perceived her struggles as related to larger gender issues, we might do so by asking a direct and simple question, such as 'Do you think self blame is a gender-based issue?' Alternatively, we might ask something more indirect and complex: 'Do you know anyone else who has trouble speaking up at times? Who? Do you know anyone else? Do you know more women or more men who have trouble speaking up? Why do you think it is that, among the people you know, more women than men have trouble speaking up?' And so on and so forth. If she didn't find our questions helpful, we would let them go.

As to your question about indicators of when we would and wouldn't want to pursue sociocultural issues, we *always* want to pursue sociocultural issues. However, we don't always pursue those issues directly and out loud. What is more important to us is that we situate our experience of people's problems within a complex and rich understanding of the discourses (such as those surrounding race, gender, class, sexual orientation, and age) that might be working to sustain those problems. Only to the extent that we ourselves can escape the clutches of sociocultural issues can we help the people who consult with us escape them. In light of this, can you see how all list-making questions are *already* sociocultural questions, in that they help people who are being storied as voiceless to have a voice?

Notes

1. This paper was first published in C. Smith & D. Nyland (eds) 1997: *Narrative Therapies with Children and Adolescents*. New York: The Guilford Press. The section 'Erica: A therapy story' is reprinted (with very minor revisions) from Freedman & Combs (1996). Copyright 1996 by Norton. Reprinted by permission.
2. Names have been changed to protect confidentiality. The family described here has granted us permission to use this material.

PART THREE

Essays:
Locating the work in context

8

Milton Erickson: Early postmodernist[1]

For a number of reasons, it feels very appropriate to be including here a paper about the work of Milton Erickson. We (JF and GC) first met each other at an Ericksonian workshop, many years ago. Early in our therapy careers we were both engrossed in Erickson's work. As it happened, when we then became interested in narrative therapy we completely misread Michael White's work. Because of our previous immersion in Ericksonian approaches, we thought Michael's questions were hypnotic (in fact, we even recall interviewing him about this!). Over time though, the clear distinctions between narrative approaches and Erickson's work became obvious to us.

Because of our longstanding interest in Ericksonian approaches to therapy, even after we had become drawn to narrative practices, we were being invited to speak at Ericksonian conferences. This chapter was written for one of those conferences. It was our way of trying to make some links between Erickson's contributions to the field of family therapy and the new postmodern narrative approaches that we were becoming increasingly engaged with and which are now our primary focus.

A couple of years ago our friends and colleagues, Melissa and Griff Griffith, were putting together an exam for the psychiatric residents they supervise in Mississippi. It was to cover some of the ideas and ways of working that constitute what we would call 'postmodern psychotherapy'. This is not an easy feat. When you have a body of knowledge that includes ideas such as 'There are no essential truths' and 'There are multiple possibilities for how to describe and classify the "reality" of any situation', a true and false test is clearly out of the question. A multiple choice test would be possible to give, but impossible to grade. Melissa and Griff settled on putting together an essay test that they believed would allow each resident to write about his or her own ideas in this arena.

Right about that time, Tom Andersen (1987), who, along with his team in the North of Norway, developed the idea of the reflecting team, and who is very interested in postmodern ideas, came to teach and consult in Mississippi at the Griffith's invitation. Melissa and Griff had been uneasy all along about having an exam, but the medical school required one. As Tom's visit grew nearer, Melissa became more and more uneasy, so much so that she buried the exam under some papers on her desk where it wouldn't come to light during Tom's visit.

But it did come to light. Somehow the test resurrected itself, and when Tom borrowed Melissa's desk to use her phone, there it was. This led to a long conversation about the exam, about Griff and Melissa's desires to be nonevaluative and collegial in their teaching, their awareness that tests of any kind in this culture don't fit with being nonevaluative and collegial, that postmodern ideas are awfully hard to test, and that there are conflicting demands in the university system. Finally, Tom said, 'When you give this test, I would ask only one thing. Could you put, at the top of the first page, 'Remember as you take this exam that there are many, many, many, right answers, and only a very few wrong ones?'

That got us to musing about our education and what it would have been like to have had such a message on an exam. In medical school and social work school we both had the impression there were right answers – and only one per question. But our continuing education, which for many years for both of us was primarily in Ericksonian approaches, was different.

I (JF) remember being at a teaching seminar in the Erickson's guesthouse some years ago. Milton Erickson primarily presented cases and told stories. Many times, although he was talking about a particular case from many years before, everyone in the room *knew* Erickson was really talking directly and specifically to him or her. We each found new associations, new thoughts, new possibilities for ourselves woven through the story Erickson was telling, although it was ostensibly about someone else. Sometimes, Erickson would work explicitly with one person, while the rest of us concentrated on learning how to do therapy as Erickson did. Simultaneously, we would have our own personal associations to, and applications of, the work he was doing. At other times, Erickson would finish presenting a case and then ask, 'What would you do?' smiling expectantly. We would banish thoughts of our personal stories as best we could and one by one suggest ways of proceeding. Then Erickson would say, 'Here's what I did', and go on to tell one of his now famous stories.

Postmodernism

A central tenet of postmodernism is that, at the social level, there is no single, essential, 'true' body of knowledge about how people, families, or societies should function. Erickson's teaching fit this idea. Here, for instance, are his (1965/1980, p.223) words from 1965:

> *The therapist's task should not be a proselytizing of the patient with his own beliefs and understandings. No patient can really understand the understandings of his therapist nor does he need them. What is needed is the development of a therapeutic situation permitting the patient to use his own thinking, his own understandings, his own emotions in the way that best fits him in his scheme of life.*

In order to describe more specifically what we mean by postmodernism, we will start by defining *modernism.* We think Roger Lowe's (1991) definition is clear and succinct:

> [modernism] ... *is used interchangeably with Enlightenment or Western thought. This form of thought insists that knowledge can be founded upon, or grounded in, absolute truth. It assumes that knowledge is 'about' something external to the knower, and can present itself objectively to the knower.*

Modernist thinkers tend to consider the scientific method as the one best way of advancing knowledge. They assume that the history of knowledge is a story of progress, of coming closer and closer to essential, foundational, generally applicable facts about the nature of a concrete and knowable universe. They tend to use metaphors based in Newtonian physics: force-counterforce, cause-effect, balance, measurement, impact, etc, DSM-III-R, with its aims of classifying all possible deviations from the norm of human mental functioning into 17 major categories and 250 or so subcategories, with the ultimate goal of finding a single specifiable cure for each distinct entity, is a paradigmatic modernist enterprise.

It seems that any modernist enterprise, when extensively pursued, begins to (if we may use a postmodernist buzzword here) deconstruct itself. Physicists, those paragons of pure science, encountered this effect during the first two decades of this century. Their quest for the fundamental building blocks of physical reality led to the description and naming of smaller and ever more numerous particles, and eventually to entities whose essential nature was unspecifiable, changing from particle to wave and back again depending on how they were measured. We all have encountered one or another reference to the relativism, uncertainty, and even metaphysical musings that surround physicists' current inquires into quarks, black holes, cold fusion, and the like.

Modernism has been slower to deconstruct itself in the field of social science, philosophy, and psychotherapy, but as our present century draws to a close, more and more psychotherapists are questioning the applicability of modernist, machine-age metaphors to our work. We are turning to *postmodernism* in one form or another for our guiding metaphors.

Postmodernism is not exactly antimodernism. Most postmodern thinkers would see the modernist worldview as one of many possible stories, one that is quite useful in pursuing criteria of predictability and control, but no more fundamentally 'true' or 'real' than many other stories about the nature of the universe. Postmodernist scholars are more interested in difference than they are in similarity. They are more interested in specific, contextualized details than they are in grand generalizations. Exceptions interest them more than rules. Clifford Geertz, a prominent postmodern voice in anthropology, has written on the importance of focusing on 'local knowledge' instead of seeking universally applicable general knowledge when trying to understand ourselves in relation to the rest of humanity. In a typical quote (1983, p.234) he says.

> ... *the world is a various place, various between lawyers and anthropologists, various between Muslims and Hindus, various between little traditions and great, various between colonial thens and nationalist nows; and much is to be gained ... by confronting that grand actuality rather than wishing it away in a haze of forceless generalities and false comforts.*

Another way of contrasting modern with postmodern thought is to say that while modernist thinkers are concerned with fact, postmodernists are concerned with meaning. In their search for and examination of meaning, postmodernists find metaphors from the humanities more useful than the modernist metaphors of physical science. 'Narrative', 'history', 'language', and 'text' are words that appear frequently in the writing of postmodernist thinkers.

As the world moves into a postmodern era (Anderson 1990; Gergen 1991), new ideas about how to do psychotherapy have begun to appear in the literature (Anderson & Goolishian 1988; Gergen 1985; Hoffman 1990; White & Epston 1990). We have been excited and energized by these ideas; they seem to fit easily with our own.

We have been surprised that many of our non-Ericksonian colleagues are not so stimulated, and even more surprised when people who are interested in postmodern ideas have difficulty applying them in therapy. We have come to believe that our background in Ericksonian ideas accounts for much of the ease and familiarity we feel in applying a postmodern worldview to psychotherapy. We think that Milton Erickson was a postmodernist before the word existed.

In the remainder of this chapter, we will consider six interrelated ideas that we believe characterize postmodern thought as it applies to psychotherapy:

1. Realities are socially constructed.
2. There are multiple possibilities for how to describe and classify the 'reality' of any situation.
3. Knowledge is *performed,* not found.
4. Knowledge is constituted through language.
5. Realities are organized and maintained through narrative.
6. There are no 'essential' truths.

There is abundant evidence that Erickson performed these knowledges long before people were talking and writing about them under the rubric of postmodernism. Let's take the ideas one at a time and see how they are exemplified in Erickson's work.

Realities are socially constructed

As the world grows smaller, people find themselves in closer contact with an increasing number of diverse cultures, and it becomes more and more obvious that 'reality isn't what it used to be'.[2]

We live a block and a half north of Devon Avenue in Chicago. The stretch of Devon due south of us is lined with Indian restaurants and stores selling saris and gold jewelry from India and Pakistan. As you proceed west on Devon, you see Jewish bakeries, kosher butcher shops, Hebrew book stores, delis, and what used to be our favorite Jewish restaurant. Also within walking distance on Devon, you can find an Islamic book store, Muslim butchers, a Thai restaurant, a Greek restaurant, a Korean restaurant, several Chinese restaurants, the Chicago Croatian Social Club, and video stores catering to Arabic and Indian clienteles. Interspersed among these stores one can find a Walgreens, a Gap clothing store, an American diner, an ice cream parlor, and various other kinds of shops that you would find most any place in North America. On Saturdays, the street is jammed with Indian families doing their weekly shopping, Hasidic men and boys on their way to and from religious services, and other people we notice less, because they look more like us.

We don't believe we should wear saris or cover our heads when we frequent Devon Avenue, but many of the people we encounter there believe that they should do one or the other. And the differences in our taken-for-granted realities don't stop at how we dress. Some of the differences that societies have constructed among themselves are so great that wars are being fought over them in other parts of the world at this very moment.

If you don't have a Devon Avenue near you, you do have a television set, and it brings you into contact with even more cultures and systems of belief. It is harder and harder to believe that the folkways that have been constructed by one's own culture are the only right and proper ways to live and believe.

We each grew up in towns largely inhabited by people of our own sociocultural-economic groups (which for each of us would not have included the other) and for each of us, the rather uniform cultures we grew up in comprised the world. But in the world we now inhabit, difference is the norm. It becomes harder and harder to deny that social realities are different in different cultures. Postmodernists believe that laws, institutions, social customs, hairstyles, and all the other things that make up the fabric of 'reality' arise through social interaction over time. In other words, we, together, construct our realities as we live them.

Erickson seems to have known about the social construction of reality from a very young age. He used to tell the story of how, when the first snowfall of the year came, he would rise especially early so that he could be the first one to school. He would take a meandering path through the fresh snow and delight in watching how the people who followed him took the same path. In later years, as we all know, he interacted socially with people to invite them into 'hypnotic realities'.[3] And on many occasions he expanded the social sphere through which new realities might be created for a particular client by engaging others to participate.

For example, he tells of Ralph, a physician he saw who had multiple problems. Erickson referred to one of the problems as his 'peculiar behavior about restaurants'. Ralph never stayed in restaurants long enough to eat a full meal, and he only frequented those with male waiters. Erickson arranged for himself and Mrs. Erickson to accompany Ralph and his wife to a restaurant for a prime rib dinner. The waitress, an old friend of the Erickson family, seated the four. The realm of social interaction through which realities could be created now included not only Ralph and Erickson, but both of their wives and the waitress. Erickson reports (Zeig 1980, p.275):

> *The waitress left us, and Ralph suddenly found that there was a clock on the wall that he could see. We waited and waited. Half an hour later the waitress showed up with four trays of salad. The waitress was very concerned. Ralph looked away and said, 'I'll take that one'. (Erickson looks away and points.)*
>
> *She said, 'You haven't even looked at it'. She used the tongs and she picked up each constituent of the salad and explained what it was. Ralph said, 'I'll take it'. She said, 'But you haven't looked at the other three*

salads'. So she had him examine all four salads twice before she let him choose his salad. Then she said, 'I have four different dressings'.

The meal continued in a drawn-out fashion, with the waitress telling jokes and eventually making Ralph clean his plate.

The next night Ralph, his wife, and daughter went back to the same restaurant and were waited on by the same well-coached waitress who was completely professional this time. From then on, Ralph was comfortable going to restaurants.

Erickson told many stories like this in which he expanded the social system to facilitate the construction of new experiential realities for the people who came to see him.

Multiple possibilities

Last summer, we had brunch at the home of some friends. When the conversation turned to the Olympics, five-year-old Ben asked us if we were rooting for the Americans. We assured him that we were and he nodded knowingly. 'That's because you're Jewish', he explained.

We think Milton Erickson would have enjoyed that moment and understood Ben's description and classification. Erickson knew a lot about the difficulties classifications can get you into and he avoided them assiduously. We think of Ben's confusion (and he *was* confused by the laughter following his statement) as a kind of postmodern dilemma: Absolute classifications just don't seem to fit in the postmodern context of so many possibilities. Ben knew his family was Jewish. They were rooting for the Americans. He drew the conclusion that Jewish people root for the Americans. Some do, but so do many African-Americans, Catholics, and other groups. There are Jews who don't root for the American teams. The possibilities are endless, and confusing – not just to five-year-olds, but to anyone trying to live by modern criteria in a postmodern world.

Erickson valued multiple possibilities. He wrote: 'There are plenty of alternatives in any situation ... When you attend a session of group therapy, what on earth are you going to see? That is what you go there for' (Erickson & Rossi 1981, p.206).

Erickson utilized the world's multiple possibilities in his therapy and teaching. He told stories of the Tarahumara Indians, the Balinese people, and other people in other places to suggest (among others) the idea that one need not be limited by the belief system that one is born into. He said, 'I had always been interested in anthropology, and I think anthropology should be something all psychotherapists should read and know about, because different ethnic groups have different ways of thinking about things' (Zeig 1980, p.119).

Knowledge is performed

Along with his celebration of multiple possibilities, the postmodern idea most clearly characterized in Erickson's work is that knowledge is *performed,* not found. It is an activity or process that we *do.*

Modernists tend to treat knowledge as if it were a commodity, something that can be uncovered, stored away, and passed intact and unchanged on to succeeding generations. Postmodernists stress the interactive and communicative aspects of knowledge. For them, it exists only in social interaction. Granted, the interaction is sometimes a conversation with oneself; but books, institutions, or traditions have meaning only when people use them. Each interaction is a new performance.

While some therapists talked with clients about their history in attempts to get to 'the root of the problem' and others hypothesized and shared those hypotheses with clients, Erickson got people to do something. He once said, 'The thing to do is to get your patient, any way you wish, any way you can, to do something' (Zeig 1980, p.143). In the act of doing, people performed knowledge. Erickson even seems to have been able to get people to perform knowledge after his physical presence had left us. The year after Erickson died, we each climbed Squaw Peak and went to the Botanical Gardens. At every Erickson Conference, we've met others who continue to do the same.

Erickson's stories and case reports are peppered with suggestions that people should 'perform knowledge' by doing something. The following is a short example from My *Voice Will Go with You* (Rosen 1982, p.127):

> *Another woman called me up and said, 'I'm ashamed to come in to see you. For the last two years I've neglected my husband, my family, my*

children. I've sat in the kitchen and eaten everything I could lay my hands on. My husband takes the children to school and brings them back. He does all the shopping and I cook and eat things. I'm grossly overweight. I don't even want you to be able to see me.'

I said, 'You want to lose the weight. You've neglected your children and your husband for two years. In that case why don't you take your children out of school; put them in the station wagon and sightsee all over Arizona, New Mexico, Utah, California, and every other cotton-pickin' place you can think of. And make your kids read brochures, historical and geographical brochures, on your sight-seeing trip. Stay in motels where you can't take charge of the kitchen. You'll be too busy looking after your kids to eat. On your husband's present income, he can join you every weekend. The family can really enjoy a vacation for a year.'

A year later she called up and said, 'I'm back to normal weight. I'm interested in my kids. I love my husband and I want to return to household duties. Do I have to do any more sight-seeing?'

I said, 'Not until you gain weight.'

Knowledge is constituted through language

Language is the medium through which we socially construct reality. By 'language' we refer to more than words. We refer to words, pictures, gestures, and the like – all the signs we use to convey meaning. In the modernist worldview, the signs of language correspond to objects and events in the 'real world'; they are passive carriers of fixed meaning. Postmodernists believe differently. They focus on how the language that we use *constitutes* our world and beliefs. Rorty (1989, p.5) puts it this way: 'Truth cannot be out there – cannot exist-independently of the human mind – because sentences cannot so exist, or be out there'.

In postmodernism, the only worlds that we can know are the worlds we describe to each other in language, and description is an active process. In agreeing on a description, we draw a distinction, and that distinction shapes subsequent distinctions, which in turn shape still other distinctions.

Here is a simple example: When I (GC) was growing up, my Uncle T. A. delighted in taking me on long walks in the woods where he would point out, name, and tell stories about the various plants and flowers we saw. Although Jill's grandparents often took her brother and her to formal gardens, they would never name flowers, but only comment on their beauty. Consequently, when we walk through the neighborhoods and parks of Chicago each spring, I see daffodils and azaleas and redbuds and bleeding hearts, and note (each and every year as if it were the first) that they bloom all at once rather than in the slow and stately progression they enjoyed in Kentucky where I grew up. Jill sees beautiful flowers. The different linguistic distinctions our families brought forth in our youth continue to constitute different knowledges of spring in our middle age.

Erickson was very aware of the constitutive power of language. Much of his work was built on the presupposition that particular language can lead to particularly altered states of consciousness. He often talked about the importance of choosing particular language in suggesting a more workable reality to a person who came to see him.

For example, when asked about seeing a couple in which the husband is an alcoholic, he said,

> *I ask him to define the problem situation for me. He'll say something like, 'I don't think I'd be an alcoholic if my wife didn't nag me all the time'. My comment to the wife is, 'I doubt if you really nag him; I expect you express your legitimate regret that he drinks excessively. And that has used a lot of your energy in the past. As he improves, what are you going to use that energy for?'*
>
> *I persuade her to wonder about that. But by putting it that way, I give the husband an opportunity to watch her to see that she uses her energy in those other areas. And he has to stop drinking so that she can have that energy to use in other areas. You always tie the two in together, but you never tell them that. When you commit her to use her time and energy elsewhere, you're committing him to give her the opportunity.* (Haley 1973, p.240)

This kind of explanation is typical of Erickson's writing and teaching and demonstrates how important he considered language to be in suggesting alternative realities.

Realities are maintained through narrative

If the distinctions that bring forth different realities are made in language, those distinctions are then circulated and remembered in stories. The central role of narrative in organizing, maintaining, and circulating knowledge of ourselves and our worlds has been stressed by many postmodern writers (e.g. Bruner 1986; Geertz 1986; Rorty 1991). Our understanding of these ideas as they apply to therapy is that people make sense of their lives through the meaning they perform on certain events. Each remembered performance constitutes a story, and the stories of individual events are strung together through time to constitute a life narrative. When life narratives offer little choice, they can be changed in therapy by the highlighting of different events or by the performing of new meaning on events, thereby constituting new narratives.

Erickson's use of stories in his teaching and psychotherapy shows that he understood the power of narrative in shaping lives. He is almost as renowned for his skilled use of stories as he is for his contributions to hypnotherapy. His well-known 'February Man' (Erickson & Rossi 1979) approach clearly illustrates how he worked actively and strategically as co-author of people's life narratives. But the most impressive illustration of Erickson's understanding of narrative's importance in shaping reality is the way that he wrote and rewrote his own life story as he lived it, performing positive meanings on what others might have experienced as adversity.

Born color blind, he took one color and made it his own. Each new purple gift from a student, colleague, or client became another incident in the complex and fascinating story of the 'Purple Sage' and all the happy associations he had involving that color. He used the knowledge he gained in his struggles with dyslexia, tone deafness, and the inability to appreciate musical rhythms to inform the inspirational and instructive stories he told others about how to persist, how to learn, and the possibility of breaking free of limiting mental sets. His nearly lifelong struggle with polio and its after-effects was a recurring theme in his 'teaching tales', and instead of framing the effects of the polio as deficits, he storied them as assets.

For instance, Rosen (1982) documents a story Erickson told about his days as a medical school professor. There was a student who became 'very withdrawn and oversensitive' after losing a leg in an auto accident. Erickson arranged for a few other students to help him stall the elevator one morning, and here's what happened:

> *On that Monday, with Jerry holding the elevator doors open and Tommy stationed at the head of the stairwell, I found the class all on the ground floor waiting for me at seven-thirty ... I said, 'What's the matter with your thumb, Sam? Is it weak? Push that elevator button.'*
>
> *He said, 'I have been'.*
>
> *I said, 'Maybe your thumb is so weak, you ought to use two thumbs'.*
>
> *He said, 'I tried that too, but that damn janitor is so worried about getting his pail and mops down, he's probably holding the elevator doors open'.*
>
> *... Finally, at five minutes of eight I turned to the student with the artificial leg and said, 'Let's us cripples hobble upstairs and leave the elevator for the able-bodied'.*
>
> *'Us cripples' started hobbling upstairs. Tommy signaled to Jerry; Sam pushed the button. The able-bodied waited for the elevator. Us cripples hobbled upstairs. At the end of the hour, that student was socializing again – with a new identity. He belonged to the professorial group: 'Us cripples'. I was a professor; I had a bad leg; he identified with me; I identified with him.* (pp.226-227)

It strikes us that, in identifying with the medical student, Erickson was writing a new chapter in his own personal narrative. He was constructing a society of professionally competent, outgoing, well-liked physicians who had the further distinction of being 'crippled', and he was placing himself squarely in the middle of that society. Later in his life, when he was confined to a wheelchair, he told his life story in such a way that it let him experience himself as an Olympic Medal winner. He told Sid Rosen (1982, p.102), 'Out of a wheelchair I win the Olympic championships all the time', and went on to recount how he had worked patiently over a number of years with Donald Lawrence to help him win two gold medals in the shot put, how he had taught the coach at Texas A & M his approach to training Lawrence, and how that coach had used his methods to train Masterson to set the first world record of 70 feet or more. It seems obvious in the telling that Erickson *had* won gold medals from his wheelchair. He was saying that if he could, so could others.

Toward the end of his life, when students began to worry aloud about Erickson's impending death, instead of joining them in their potentially pessimistic narratives, he told stories of the longevity and optimism of his parents. We believe that these stories served an inspirational purpose for Erickson's students and for Erickson himself, advancing the social construction of the mindset that led him to say, 'I have no intention of dying. In fact, that will be the last thing I do!' (Rosen 1982, p.167)

There are no essential truths

If realities are socially constructed, and if knowledge is performed and constituted through language, it follows that, at least at the social level, truth is somewhat fluid and negotiable; there are no essential truths. For instance, the modernist idea of norms, such as criteria for mental health or developmental stages, is still dominant in our culture. Many people compare themselves to norms with the belief that in so doing they will discover some essential truth about themselves. Looking through a postmodernist lens, we see such concepts as stories about ways of being, not as descriptions of essential truth.

While modernists speak as if they believe in a deep, real, or essential self, postmodernists believe that self-knowledge is performed and constituted through language and maintained through narrative. There are multiple possibilities for how people constitute themselves through social interaction. Certainly, particular possibilities are preferred by particular people and particular cultures, but none represent essences.

This does not mean that 'anything goes'. Tradition, personal history, and 'common sense' constrain us, blinding us to certain possibilities and leading us to see others as desirable. Saying that values are socially constructed does not mean that all values should be tossed out the window or that all societies construct equally useful values. However, it does mean that we can strive for the awareness of the subjectivity of our worldviews and cultivate humility in the face of beliefs that conflict with our own.

Even before we encountered the essential/constructed distinction and distinguished ourselves as constructionists, our immersion in Erickson's teachings led us to agree with Erickson's words (Erickson & Rossi 1979, pp.233-234):

> *Psychotherapists cannot depend upon general routines or standardized procedures to be applied indiscriminately to all their patients. Psychotherapy is not the mere application of truths and principles supposedly discovered by academicians in controlled laboratory experiments. Each psyotherapeutic encounter is unique and requires fresh creative effort on the part of both therapist and patient to discover the principles and means of achieving a therapeutic outcome.*

As early as the '30s Erickson (1930/1980, p.482) was writing:

> *Properly, it* [therapy] *is not a matter of advancing particular schools of thought or of attempting to substantiate interpretive psychological theories, but simply a task of appraising a patient's problem or problems in terms of the reality in which the patient lives and in the terms of the realities of the patient's continuing future as he or she may reasonably hope for it to be.*

Because they don't believe in essential truths, postmodernists prefer qualitative research – ethnography, narrative descriptions, case histories, and the like – over quantitative research. Erickson (1953, p.2), always ahead of his time, had this to say back in 1953:

> *... single instances often illustrate clearly and vividly aspects and facts of general configurations, trends and patterns. Rather than proof of specific ideas, an illustration or portrayal of possibilities is often the proper goal of experimental work.*

We believe that Erickson was intensely curious about the 'local knowledge' of each new person be met, and he knew that such knowledge had to be, must be, different in many ways from anyone else's knowledge. He celebrated that difference and built his way of working around it. He wrote about cases, about specific people at specific moments in their lives, not about theory and not about essential, overarching truth – which brings us to the title of this volume, 'Ericksonian Methods: The Essence of the Story'.

Is there an essence to his story? Many people, ourselves (Combs & Freedman 1990) included, having studied Erickson's work through our own filters, have drawn distinctions that we thought captured some essence or other of Erickson's work. These methods, patterns, techniques, guidelines, approaches, or whatever we called them have been useful in developing our psychotherapeutic skills. But none of us has ever captured the essence of Erickson's story. Margaret Mead (1977) may have come close when she wrote, 'It can be firmly said that Milton Erickson never solves a problem in an old way if he can think of a new way – and he usually can' (pp.4-5). We believe the essence of the story is that there is no essence.[4]

Each one of us, each community of us as we strive to apply Ericksonian ideas in our daily work, constitutes a particular local knowledge, an embodied enactment, of Erickson's story. And each embodied enactment is unique. Personally, we are glad to have Erickson's examples to emulate. But our every attempt at copying his methods turns out different. As Geertz (1986, p.380) puts it, 'It is the copying that originates'.

Try as we might, we cannot replicate Erickson's work, nor, we believe, would he want us to. He celebrated the uniqueness of his students as well as that of his clients, urging them to do things their own way. Remember what Tom Andersen said, 'There are many, many, many right answers and only a very few wrong ones'.

Notes

1. This paper was originally published in Zeig, J. 1994: *Ericksonian Methods: the essence of the story*. New York: Brunner/Mazel.
2. This is the title of W.T. Andersen's (1990) popular book about postmodern culture.
3. See the book of the same title by Erickson, Rossi, & Rossi (1976).
4. In the discussion following our presentation of this paper, Michael Rousell PhD, from Alberta, Canada, made a comment that we found intriguing. He said that if 'realities are organized and maintained through narrative, which is what we appear to do, ever since we've been talking about Erickson we've been talking about his story and maintaining him through story. So maybe the essence of the story is the story of his essence.'

9

Narrative intentions[1]

One of the many aspects of narrative practice that first appealed to us was the way in which its intentions depart from the strategic tradition. Within narrative practice the therapist's role is not one of creating strategies to make change occur in other people's relationships. Rather than being informed by an ethic of control, narrative practice is instead informed by an ethic of collaboration and this makes possible entirely different relationships between therapists and those who consult them. The groundwork for this orientation to therapy was in some ways provided by the work of Gianfranco Cecchin (1987) whose influential work on curiosity provided impetus towards a therapy of questioning rather than intervening.

In beginning to teach narrative ideas, what soon became clear to us was the need to clarify some of the intentions that inform which questions to ask, when. We realised that when we did not do this, some of the people who had come for training would simply ask questions because they were curious about the answers, rather than because they had any map or idea as to how such questions might create space for the person involved to address the reasons they had sought therapy.

So, we began to articulate more clearly how, within a narrative approach, the reason we ask questions is to invite people to story their experience and to do so in relation to both problematic and alternative stories in their lives. By generating richer description of the alternative stories of people's lives they become more available and easier to perform, and this in turn can lead to significant positive effects on people's lives. The following paper, 'Narrative Intentions', was written to explain this.

At the same time, I (Gene) was in the midst of a number of discussions with therapists associated with Harry Goolishian and Harlene Anderson's highly respected Houston-Galveston Institute. These were discussions about the role of the therapist, and whether our intention should be simply to listen and to expand the options for conversation and dialogue, or whether our role is to ask questions that more deliberately invite the richer description of alternative stories. This is a good conversation and one that continues to some extent in the broader family therapy field. This paper on 'Narrative Intentions' was one way of clarifying our beliefs about the role we wish to play as therapists.

When we present examples of our work to other therapists they often ask about particular moments in the therapy: 'How did you know to ask that?' or, 'Why did you do that?' While there are many different ways to answer such a question, we believe that *narrative intentions* are a major influence on the moment-by-moment choices we make in working with people.

In the pages of this book[2], although the authors have come together because of shared assumptions and values, one can find various sets of intentions. For example, some therapists intend to engage in conversations through which solutions will be constructed. Others intend to converse in ways that focus on the meaning of what people say, believing that a careful focus on meaning cannot help but engender the dissolution of old meanings as new ones emerge. While our work is informed by many of the intentions one can find in this book, our central intention is to collaborate with people in developing new narratives about themselves and the worlds they inhabit.

A guiding metaphor, such as narrative, is no small matter. We recently presented a videotape of a small segment of our work to a group of colleagues, each of whom uses a different model of therapy. To our way of thinking, what happened on the tape was that a couple, Jan and Arthur, came to therapy with their lives situated in a story of misunderstanding and disappointment. They described several incidents in which misunderstanding and disappointment had come between them. However, they also mentioned in an offhand way a task they had completed together. We talked with them about this achievement, asking how they had accomplished it and what it meant about them that they could accomplish it. They described the process they used in working together and agreed that it showed they could cooperate and even be creative with each other. We asked about other times in their relationship when they had cooperated and been creative with each other, and they recounted several such incidents. We wondered what difference it would make to know that they could accomplish things through cooperation and do so creatively. They said it would mean that not only could they work together to deal with misunderstandings, but they also could look forward to doing anything they decided to do together. When we fast forwarded to the end of the tape, the two were excitedly recounting incidents in which they had worked together and planning shared projects for the future.

To our way of thinking, they had begun to 'restory' their relationship. What started as a story of misunderstanding and disappointment was becoming a story of cooperation and creativity. When we showed this tape excerpt, we expected that our colleagues would see and hear the kinds of things we have just described.

The first person to comment said, 'I don't know what to make of your tape, I'm used to helping people understand problems and you hardly talked about the problem at all. I kept waiting to get back to the problem.'

Several people joined in a discussion of what the problem 'really' was. The problems they saw did not have to do with stories of misunderstanding and disappointment but with a variety of other things such as legacies from families of origin, life-cycle phases, and diagnostic categories.

This discussion was interrupted by another colleague who said, 'I thought there was quite a lot of talk about the problem, but no goals were set. I was confused about how you could decide on a direction without setting goals.'

Later, as the two of us discussed the experience, we agreed that we did not recognize our work in their comments. Our colleagues, guided by different metaphors, did not see or hear the tape as we did. We, in turn, did not see or hear what they did. Luigi Boscolo once told us, 'You can only see what you see'. We would add that the metaphors that guide one's intentions shape both what one sees and what one does.

We come to narrative therapy by way of the world of Ericksonian therapy (see, e.g. Combs & Freedman 1990). In my (JF) early training in Ericksonian approaches, I remember being taught the presupposition that everyone has all the resources he or she needs to reach his or her goals. One of the people in the training program had a hard time believing this idea in relation to some of the people at the agency where he worked. He explained his difficulty to the trainer and asked if the presupposition was really true in every case. The trainer considered the question for a moment and then answered, 'I don't know if it's true or not. What I do know is that I get farther with people if I believe it.'

The narrative analogy, like any other map or model, is a metaphor. Our intention in this paper is not to establish it as a 'right' or 'true' map for understanding people's experience or for guiding our intentions in psychotherapy. What we hope to illustrate is how far we get and in what directions we go when we let this particular metaphor guide our intentions.[3]

We will give an overview of our intentions and the actions that flow from them. Then we will describe the work we undertook with a particular person and comment on how narrative intentions influenced our contributions to that work.

A narrative map and how it shapes our intentions

We base our therapy on the notion that people make meaning of their lives by organizing key events into stories, which they then incorporate into a larger life narrative (E. Bruner 1986; J. Bruner 1986; Geertz 1986; White & Epston 1990). Such stories are social constructs (Gergen 1985; Hoffman 1990), arrived at through interaction and experience with other people in a particular historical-cultural context. Furthermore, as Michael White (1991, p. 28) writes:

> *Not only do these stories determine the meaning that persons give to experience, ... but these stories also largely determine which aspects of experience persons select out for expression. And, as well, inasmuch as action is prefigured on meaning-making, these stories determine real effects in terms of the shaping of persons' lives.*

People who come to therapy can be viewed as living in stories where choice is restricted and available options are painful or unfulfilling. Our work involves facilitating experience of new stories – life narratives that are more empowering, more satisfying, and give hope for better futures.

This narrative metaphor is a constant influence on what we notice, what we are most interested in, the kinds of questions we ask, and the ideas that we have during therapy. When people experience themselves as inhabiting more meaningful stories, their ongoing perceptions, choices, and behavior will change more or less automatically. For this reason, we focus on expanding and enriching meaning more than on encouraging new behavior.

Our role in this process mainly involves listening and asking questions. This helps us stay as much as possible in a position of 'not knowing' (Anderson & Goolishian 1990). Asking questions rather than making interpretive, diagnostic, or interventive statements invites people to clarify and redirect our understanding at each turn of the conversation.

Although this chapter focuses on what therapists think and do, we in no sense want to imply that what therapists think and do is the most important aspect of what happens in therapy. It is simply the side for which we bear responsibility. Our intention is to engage in collaborative, horizontal relationships in which people choose stories they prefer and make their own meanings about those preferred stories. White & Epston (1990) describe it this way:

> *As a general rule, persons cannot see unique possibilities for their lives if others are standing in front of them, blocking their view ...*
>
> *Supporting persons from behind is not problematic in this way. The therapist can achieve this position in a general sense by working to identify unique outcomes and by directly engaging the person in the performance of new meanings around these. Thus, the person is encouraged to be the privileged author of the new story.* (pp.148-149)

Deconstructive listening

Narrative intentions lead us to listen to what people tell us as stories (therefore, not as chief complaints, information to be 'gathered', matrices within which resources are embedded, lists of symptoms from which to make diagnoses, surface hints about what the core problem 'really' is, or anything else except stories). Since each person has lived experience that does not fit with the problem-saturated story that he or she has brought to therapy, it is tempting to immediately begin asking about such exceptional experience. However, doing so can lead people to feel that the seriousness of their problems is not understood or that their versions of reality are not valued. Listening carefully to people's stories and striving to understand their experience helps both to develop trust and rapport and to have some ideas about the particular constraints their stories carry.

As important as it is to listen to problem-saturated stories, it is even more important not to let our listening reify undesired meanings. We have come to refer to the special kind of listening required for accepting and striving to understand problem-saturated stories without reifying them as *deconstructing listening.*

In academic circles, the word 'deconstruction' immediately brings to mind the work of Jacques Derrida (e.g. 1988), which explores, among other things, the slipperiness of meaning, examining and illustrating how the meaning of any symbol, word, or text is inextricably bound up in its context. Deconstructionists believe that it is fruitless to search for the 'real' meaning of any text. Any narrative is full of gaps and ambiguities. Deconstructionist scholars focus on these gaps and ambiguities to show that the officially sanctioned or generally accepted meaning of a given text is but one of a great number of possible meanings.

Listening deconstructively to people's stories requires situating oneself in the belief that the stories people tell have many possible meanings and that the meaning a listener makes is often not exactly the same as the meaning that the speaker has intended. This belief leads us to listen for gaps and ambiguities in meaning and, when we hear them, either to ask people to fill in details or to tell them the meaning we are hearing and ask how it fits with their intended meaning.

Listening deconstructively begins with the 'not-knowing' attitude that we have already mentioned. When therapists successfully cultivate a not-knowing attitude, therapy is conducted in an atmosphere of wondering, of, 'What if ...?' or, 'Could it be that ...?' This is very different from therapy conducted in an atmosphere of searching for clues to the one correct diagnosis or offering interpretations of the deep truth.

The dominant stories in Western culture still value decisiveness, action, and certitude. In our experience, this makes it difficult for therapists to stay in a not-knowing position. However, at least until the dominant stories change, it also makes it more likely that therapists who work in an atmosphere of not knowing will provide novel experiences for the people with whom they work. Such an atmosphere invites people to entertain the belief that they are the experts in regard to their life stories.

Our not knowing is colored by two beliefs or attitudes that we find compellingly useful in inviting people to deconstruct unsatisfying life narratives. The first of these is that life narratives are constructed bit by bit over time by people in interaction with other people; that is, they are *socially constructed* (Berger & Luckmann 1966; Gergen 1985). This belief leads us to interact with people in ways that invite them to relate to their life narratives not as passively received facts, but as actively constructed stories. Such interaction begins to deconstruct the 'factity' of their narratives.

The second belief that colors our not knowing is Michael White's idea (1987, 1989; see also Tomm 1989) that people are separate from their problems; that is, people are not the problem but the problem is the problem. Thus, when listening to people's descriptions of themselves or each other, we ask ourselves, 'What is the problem that leads these people to behave in this way or have this kind of experience?' By 'problem' we are not referring to a diagnostic category, but to an externalized and objectified idea, process, or emotion. That is, when a person says something such as, 'I'm not a very good person. I seem to always do things wrong', we might begin to wonder if guilt is coloring his or her view of himself or herself. Thus, the person is invited to perceive 'guilt' rather than his or her 'self' as the problem. With our question, an *externalizing conversation* (White 1991) is initiated about what he or she finds problematic.

As people tell their stories, we interrupt at intervals to summarize our understanding of their stories so that they can help us track their meaning and so that they can tell us if the meaning we are making fits for them. In responding to our questions and comments, people must examine their old stories in new ways. The beliefs and attitudes that we listen with create a new context, and in this new context, meanings are different. We listen with a thoughtfulness about what constructions are being made as we try to understand each other. As we perceive a possible new construction emerging, we ask if it is a fitting and helpful way of thinking about the story and we make adjustments in accordance with people's answers. Most of this process occurs automatically and subliminally as a result of our beliefs about narrative and social constructionism. It is not a didactic or intellectual process; we rarely, if ever, talk directly about social constructionism or externalization. Instead, we strive to listen closely and carefully with an attitude that is solidly grounded in these notions. When we listen with this attitude we find that, in the act of telling us their 'old stories', people begin to view those stories as social constructions that are not fixed truths and, we hope, to entertain the idea that other stories that are just as true might suit them better.

Deconstructive questioning

So far, deconstruction has been discussed as something that is a natural and inevitable by-product of our efforts to understand people's life stories through a narrative/social constructionist filter. The primary intention of our questions has been to gain understanding of people's problem-saturated narratives. At some point, usually when it seems that a certain degree of trust and mutual understanding has been achieved, we begin to ask questions of a more purposefully interventive nature. Our intention shifts from that *of understanding* people's problem-saturated stories to that of *deconstructing* those stories.

Questions with a deconstructive intent invite people to see their stories from a different perspective, to notice how they are constructed (or *that* they are constructed), to note their limits, or to discover that there are other possible narratives. To accomplish this, inquiry is directed toward the beliefs, practices, and feelings that support a narrative or develop from it.

For example, in the tape of Jan and Arthur, one of us (GC) asked this question: 'Has disappointment kept you from responding to some things and encouraged you to respond strongly to others?' My intention in asking this question was to invite the couple to consider how the story of disappointment may have directed their attention toward disappointing events. If they adopted this view, they would begin to see how stories of disappointment construct experiences of disappointment, and to entertain the possibility of constructing other stories. Jan and Arthur, in fact, did decide that the constructions they were making were not in their best interest. They then began to identify and make meaning of other, previously unstoried, events.

Listening for and asking about openings

Saying that people make meaning of their lives by organizing selected events into stories oversimplifies the situation. People are born into stories; their social and historical contexts constantly invite them to story certain events and leave others unstoried. As a narrative takes shape, it powerfully influences the selections a person makes about what further events should be storied. The countless experiences, actions, and thoughts that remain unstoried are potential 'unique outcomes' (White 1988, 1989), which present possible openings into alternative stories. Narrative intentions lead us to listen attentively for such openings (we are using 'listen' broadly here, as an activity for eyes as well as ears) and even to inquire directly about their existence.

In the example of Jan and Arthur, the offhand remark that they had completed a task together was an opening that led to an alternative story of cooperation and creativity. If they had not mentioned this event or if the meaning they found in it did not seem to open onto a story that they preferred, we could have asked, 'Have there been times that you have been able to keep misunderstanding and disappointment from dominating your relationship?' or,

'When was a time that you felt understood by each other?' Either of these questions might have led to an opening, which in turn might have led to an alternative story.

Developing new stories

All the previous discussion of listening and questioning sets the stage for our central intention, which is to assist people in developing new stories. Once problem-saturated stories are understood as social constructions, different, more fruitful constructions can be privileged. Unique outcomes constitute openings that, through questions and discussion, can be developed into new stories. Once a unique outcome is 'storied' in a meaningful way, its precursors can be found and included in the narrative and its future can be speculated on and included in the narrative. The new meanings embodied in the emerging story can support new perceptions and behaviors, which will affect other people, whose reactions can also become part of the ever expanding narrative.

More specifically, when possible openings are perceived, we ask questions that invite people to develop them into alternative stories. Initially, we ask questions such as, 'Does this interest you?' 'Did that surprise you?' 'Is this something that you want more of in your life?' or, 'Do you think this is a good thing or a bad thing?' Questions like these invite people to consider whether something that we see as a possible opening is really new for them and whether it opens in a direction that they prefer over the direction of the problem story. Our questions are invitations, not directives. We know that we want to lead the conversation in the direction of new stories, but we want to stay in a posture of genuinely not knowing what will constitute a meaningful opening or exactly where that opening will lead. Therefore, it is important to notice quickly when people decline invitations, and to listen until openings that interest them occur. To do otherwise involves the risk of becoming yet another source of oppressive restraint.

If the opening seems to be a preferred one, we will ask questions to encourage the development of an alternative story. We do not have a formula to follow in this process. We do keep in mind that stories involve events that happen through time in particular contexts and that they usually include several people. Also, a big part of what stories these events is that people 'perform meaning' (Myerhoff 1986; White 1991; White & Epston 1990) on them; that is, they attribute meaning to them and treat them as important. In the following sections, examples are given of some of the different kinds of questions that are useful in restorying. For more thorough accounts of questions that can be used in the re-authoring process, see White (1988) and Freedman and Combs (1993).

Asking how

Once an opening that is both novel and preferred has been negotiated, we want to know how the person brought that opening about. Questions like, 'How did you do that?', 'What did you do that led you to feel this new feeling?' and, 'How did you arrive at this different way of perceiving the situation?' are useful in this regard. Answers to such questions almost always come in the form of stories.[4] Sometimes people give such full answers to these questions that no further work at story development seems necessary for that particular opening.

When we ask 'how' we are implicitly inviting people to join us in a powerful presupposition: that they have *personal agency* in effecting unique outcomes. Narratives without such a sense of agency tend to be narratives of powerlessness and oppression, so we work to co-author narratives in which people experience themselves as capable, creative, and effective. However, if a person clearly indicates a sense of passivity in regard to a particular unique outcome, that perception can be accepted and used to explore how the problematic story promotes such a sense of passivity and possibly set the stage for its deconstruction.

Detail

Sometimes a person will clearly indicate that an opening is interesting, but will find 'how' questions difficult to answer. In such cases, one can ask for more details: 'What happened just before that?' 'What happened next?' 'Where were you exactly?' 'Who else was there?' 'What did you say?' 'What did they say?' 'How did it feel to do that?' 'What were you thinking as it happened?'

'Who was the first person you told about the incident?' Our intention here is to invite the elaboration of enough detail (particularities of action, character, mood, setting, etc.) for the singular event of the opening to become an experientially vivid story.

Performing meaning

As a story begins to unfold on what White (1988), following Jerome Bruner (1986), calls the 'landscape of action', it is useful to ask questions that direct people's attention to the 'landscape of consciousness'. Bruner has discussed how the interplay between these 'dual landscapes' invites empathic and experiential involvement in the lives and minds of the characters in a story. We ask what we (Freedman & Combs 1993) call *meaning questions,* with the intention of inviting people to enter the thoughts, feelings, and beliefs engendered by the actions they have recounted. Examples of meaning questions include: 'What do you make of that?' 'What does that tell you about your relationship?' 'What did you learn from that experience?' and, 'What does that mean to you now?' Again, asking questions out of curiosity rather than out of a push for therapist-preferred meanings creates a context in which the people who have sought our assistance have the greater voice in the re-authoring process.

Extending the story in time

Just as Jan and Arthur did not develop the story of their relationship as one of misunderstanding and disappointment from a single incident, the unique outcome of completing a task together was only an opening for an alternative story, not a whole new narrative in and of itself. Connecting that bit of story with others eventually did constitute a new narrative.

Similarly, people are almost always invited to consider the story developed around any particular opening within a broader flow of time. Until such stories are linked into narratives with a past, present, and future (Boscolo & Bertrando 1992), they are in danger of easily being overshadowed by old, dominant stories.

One way to facilitate the incorporation of a number of stories into the same flow of time is by linking newly storied events to related events that have not yet been storied. One might attempt this by asking, 'Was there another time, farther in the past, that this incident reminds you of?' or, 'At what stage in your previous history were you most aware of this quality that you are rediscovering in yourself now?' Often, such a question will trigger a memory that can be developed into another bit of new story. When the person connects the stories of the two incidents, it is not uncommon for still other related incidents to spring to mind. As these 'preferred' stories are strung together on the time line of a single life narrative, that narrative cannot help but change in ways that the client prefers.

We can also ask how a particular bit of new story influences a person's ideas about the future. Questions like, 'How does this incident change your ideas about what might happen in your relationship over the next week?' and, 'Now that you know this, what's the next step?' invite people to alter their plans and expectations so that they are more in line with the emerging story. Such alterations increase the likelihood of new life events that will constitute lived experience of the new story. Meaning can be performed on these new life events in future sessions.

Clinical example

We would like to say at the outset that while 'Jessica' quickly achieved spectacular results, our experience with people is often less dramatic. This story was chosen because in addition to being dramatic, it is very clear, straightforward, and easy to follow. Remember, however, that what follows is a much simplified and 'cleaned-up' report that is intentionally edited and annotated to emphasize how narrative intentions on the part of the therapist contributed to a satisfying outcome for Jessica. In this way it is a lot like the kind of 'new story' we invite people to construct for themselves. At the time I (JF) met Jessica she had just completed several years of therapy. She felt that her therapist[5] had been helpful and supportive, but she had not perceived any progress for a number of months and had come to believe that 'it had gone as far as it could go'. Within a few months of that ending Jessica heard me give a talk on sexual abuse, which gave her hope that maybe she could go farther. She called me to set up an appointment, explaining that she felt stuck and hoped that I would see her even though she lived three hours away and did not know how often she could come to see me. Our usual practice in setting appointments is to ask people at the end of each session if and when they would like to have another appointment. In Jessica's situation, distance necessitated less frequent sessions than she would have chosen otherwise. One of the ways we accommodated the distance was by incorporating the possibility of brief phone calls between sessions.

The first session

Jessica was the head nurse for the emergency room of the only hospital in a medium-sized city in southern Illinois. She lived alone in a farmhouse on the edge of town, had a sizeable circle of female friends, and enjoyed participating in sports.[6]

In the first session, Jessica told me that she was 35 years old and had never had a romantic relationship. She described growing up in a family where women were treated as the property of men. Her father and uncle touched her, her mother, and her sister in any way they liked at any time they liked. The touching was often rough and often sexual, including having her breast or crotch grabbed while she was helping with kitchen chores and being forced into sexual contact with one man while another looked on.

I asked Jessica what the effects of this abuse were on her, both in the past, as a child, and now, as an adult. She said that, as a child, the abuse brought forth feelings of fear, insecurity, confusion, helplessness, and isolation. She elaborated on these themes in some detail. The effects on her as an adult were an inability to engage in a romantic relationship, difficulty in friendships, and feelings of worthlessness. Again, she gave examples of how these played out in her life.

I wondered, and asked aloud, how she had moved from a childhood of fear, insecurity, confusion, helplessness, and isolation to the different place that she now inhabited. She helped me understand how the present effects (inability to engage in a romantic relationship, difficulty in friendships, and feelings of worthlessness) were the remnants of earlier difficulties. She explained that the feelings of worthlessness were limited to social situations. In fact, it turned out that all the effects of abuse had become contextualized and no longer took over her life as they had when she was a child.

Jessica had a Master's degree, and she described her job as head nurse as a good one, which she had held for a number of years. I asked her what it would have meant to her if she had been able to see these things in her future when she was a child. She said that she would have realized that the fear and related feelings were not inherent truths about her. If they were, she would not have been able to accomplish as much as she had professionally. I was very interested in how she had been able to stand up to the effects of the abuse over the years and determine her own career. I hoped we would be able to talk more about this.

Jessica commented that, now that she thought about it, her accomplishments really were remarkable, especially because no one else in her family had ever gone to college or become a professional.

Commentary

In the beginning, we listen to people's existing narratives. As we listen, we orient ourselves to their experiential worlds. The intimate and graphic details that Jessica volunteers are evidence that a relationship of trust and mutual respect is developing. Only as such evidence is perceived do we feel comfortable about inviting much in the way of new story. For people with stories like Jessica's, attempting to change things right away can be experienced as yet one more violation and disqualification by a powerful other. At the same time, it is important to be careful not to reify or replicate the abuse by becoming voyeuristically involved and pushing for more detail than the person freely and comfortably gives (Durrant & Kowalski 1990).

From the beginning of therapy, we listen deconstructively. For instance, Jessica did not use the words, 'the property of men', but our feminist values lead us to hear stories like hers in these terms and to use such terms in therapy as we summarize our understanding of the emerging narrative. When constructions like these are offered in the conversation, people examine their own way of constructing the situation in the light of our constructions (Kamsler 1990). This kind of comparison is a basic act of deconstruction.

Inquiring about the effects of the abuse is a more active form of deconstructive listening. Jessica is invited to tell a story about 'having been affected by abuse' rather than a story about 'being an abused person'. When Jessica accepts this invitation, she can experience abuse less as a part of her identity and more as a separate entity with which she can struggle. When she compares the past with the present effects of the abuse, Jessica presents what seems like an opening. Using White's (1987) notion of 'collapsing time', which involves such comparisons, helped bring forth this opening.

Jessica was asked a 'how' question (How had she moved from a childhood of fear, insecurity, confusion, helplessness, and isolation to the different place that she now inhabited?) which invited her to consider her influence in altering the effects of the abuse. Her response indicated that she was interested in this opening and that she had already developed some new story around it, so she was asked a 'meaning question' (What would it have meant to her if she had been able to see these things in her future when she was a child?), which invited her to reflect on the meaning of her childhood fears and the like, in the light of the alternative story that she was developing.

Jessica's response to the meaning question presented another opening, which prompted another 'how' question (How had she been able to stand up to the effects of the abuse over the years and determine her own career?), asked in a way that implied it could be explored further in the next session and that invited Jessica to develop more new story between sessions. At the end of the session, Jessica began to reflect on her achievements as 'remarkable' and, therefore, to story herself as a remarkable person.

The second session

At the second session, which we had scheduled for six weeks later, Jessica said she now realized that she was no longer the child that she once had been, and that life was very different for her as an autonomous adult than it had been for her as a dependent child. Now, she felt ready to get married and raise a family. She wanted to work on smiling, because people kept telling her to smile.

I asked if it would be all right to slow things down a little in the session so that I could keep up with her. When she agreed, I asked her how she had come to this realization that she was no longer the child she once had been. She went over some of the same ground as she had in the first session, this time going into more detail about the differences in her past and present experience. This time, she had more ideas about things she had done to create an identity for herself instead of letting the effects of the abuse create her identity. Experiences at school, a place where she excelled, got positive comments, and was treated with fairness, were very important sources of self-knowledge that she used in creating her identity. These experiences of mastery and of being treated as a person rather than as property nurtured a secret part of her. Over time, she was able to develop that part, and it enabled her to stand up to the effects of the abuse and limit their area of influence.

I asked her what the fact that she had accomplished all this meant about her. With some hesitation, looking away from me, she said it meant that she was smart and tough. I said I understood that people outside of her family did not know about her home situation, but I wondered if they had known, who might have predicted that she would be able to stand up to the effects of the abuse and not let it take over her life. She said that teachers and kids at school knew she was smart and tough. Had they known about her situation at home, they would probably have predicted that she would find a way to oppose the abuse and take her life back for herself. Her previous therapist also recognized these qualities in her.

I then wondered aloud, 'If we look back over the years at how you have used your strength and intelligence to take charge of your life – you got an education, became a head nurse, and found ways to limit the effects of the abuse – is this readiness to get married that you are talking about the next step?' She thought maybe it was. As we began to talk about what that meant, Jessica acknowledged that it was different to think of herself as someone who could have an intimate life with someone else. Not only was she smart and tough, but now she could begin to imagine herself having warm and tender feelings and connecting with another person, In fact, in her previous therapy, she had felt connected to her therapist and had a variety of pleasant feelings toward her. She could now see that relationship as preparation for other relationships. In friendships with women, she had also experienced some positive feelings and connection, even though these relationships were often rocky.

As we talked more about the possibility of moving into the realm of romantic relationship, we discovered that simply thinking about herself as someone who could operate in that realm was an important step in taking her life back from the effects of the abuse. Because the effects of the abuse had held her social life hostage for so long, there were probably a number of important social experiences that the effects had robbed her of until now. For example, Jessica did not really think of men as people, so making friends with a man might be an important step, and now she knew that her intelligence could help her pick a safe man for the project.

Commentary

Jessica has developed a lot of new story between sessions. She is perceiving herself differently and identifying new and ambitious goals for herself. At times like this, it is important to develop as rich, detailed, and meaningful a story as possible. It is also important to invite, when possible, enhancement of the 'personal agency' aspects of the emerging story (Adams-Westcott, Dafforn & Sterne 1993). Here, this is accomplished by asking 'how' in a way that presupposes personal agency – how she came to the realization that she was no longer the child she had once been.

A wonderful and richly detailed story of standing up to the effects of abuse and creating an identity for herself comes forth in response to the question. This story was always a possible part of Jessica's life narrative, but, until the last six weeks, the events from which it is assembled had been lying around disconnected and gathering dust in seldom-visited memories.

In response to another meaning question (What does the fact that she has accomplished all this mean about her?), Jessica begins to own 'smart' and 'tough' as real and prominent personal attributes supported by her life narrative. As the interchange continues, Jessica is invited to flesh out the story of how she has been smart and tough enough to stand up to the effects of the abuse. Her attention is directed toward other people who appreciate these qualities and abilities in her. Jessica identifies several members of her 'supporting cast', and realizes that the story that she is only now discovering has already been circulated in her past and present social world. All these people genuinely believe her to be smart and tough, and now that she appreciates their knowledge, it will be much harder for the old narrative of fear, insecurity, confusion, helplessness, and isolation to take over.

Before we adopted a narrative map, we worked to help people identify 'resources' from non-problematic life contexts, and to use those resources in problematic contexts. It was quite common for us to search through past experiences for these resources. However, we thought of the resources as states of consciousness and used past experiences only as a way to help people access resourceful states. We made little effort to connect experiences and states through time. Now we think of such experiences as important life events that, when given prominence in a person's life narrative, will alter the meaning of that narrative in satisfying ways. This leads us to expend much more energy on reviewing the past and less energy on helping people 'access states'.

With the question about 'the next step', the idea of wanting a romantic relationship, which Jessica voiced in therapy, is brought up for possible inclusion in the narrative. She is invited to consolidate the developing new story and extend it into the future. She responds by identifying additional personal characteristics and realizing that they are already part of who she has been and will be, thus continuing to revise her life narrative.

In the ensuing conversation, externalizing language is used to invite Jessica to view her narrative as one in which her romantic life has been held hostage by the effects of the abuse. Since she is already, at this point, storying herself as smart, tough, and at least a little experienced in warm and tender relationships, rescuing her romantic life may *no longer* seem such a daunting job.

The third session

In the third session, one month later, Jessica was taken over by distress about events in one of her friendships. In her estimation, a close woman friend often treated her badly – criticizing her, refusing to talk to her – but Jessica had chosen so far to spend time with her anyway. It was after the most recent bout of these incidents that the distress had taken over. The belief that other people they both knew sided with her friend made the distress even stronger.

I wondered aloud if Jessica's implied desire to do something different with this friendship was a part of the previously identified project of rescuing her social life from the effects of the abuse. Considering it in this light, Jessica thought that the way she had been up to now in the relationship was influenced by the effects of the abuse, but now she felt this way of being was intolerable. I reminded her of the personal qualities she had owned more closely – strength, intelligence, ability to have warm and tender feelings, ability to connect – and wondered how these might be useful in this problematic relationship.

She decided to put her professional self – the part of her that had done well at school and work, and whose intelligence and strength she trusted – in charge of setting limits and deciding what she should do to take care of herself in this relationship. I asked if she thought doing this would constitute progress toward being more secure in other relationships. She thought it would.

Commentary

'Taken over by distress' is an externalizing construction. As always, it is important to notice whether or not this construction fits for Jessica. In this case, it seems to.

Jessica is invited to incorporate the current crisis into the narrative she began to build over the course of her first two sessions, a story in which she is a person with certain personal characteristics who is engaged in a project of rescuing her social life from the effects of abuse. In response to this invitation, Jessica comes up with a plan for how to proceed in the problematic relationship. Again, narrative intentions make us want to incorporate significant events into the overall flow of past, present, and future that constitutes a person's life narrative. As she successfully resolves the current crisis, it will become a significant chapter in the story of how she rescued her social life from the effects of abuse.

The fourth session

Jessica came to the fourth session (again, one month later) taken over by distress and also by confusion about her relationship with this same friend. She had consistently used her intelligence and strength in setting limits and making decisions. Her friend had countered with criticism and name calling. This brought forth self-doubt for Jessica. She particularly began to experience doubt about whether it was possible for her to be healthy, normal, or playful.

I wondered out loud if there were times when she had been sure of her ability to be 'healthy', 'normal', and 'playful', even for a moment. With some encouragement, Jessica remembered learning a song at school. Her grandmother, who lived out of town, was visiting, and when Jessica came home from school that day her grandmother was there alone. Jessica remembered sitting on her grandmother's lap and teaching her the song; her grandmother looked into her eyes, smiled, and sang with Jessica, clearly enjoying her company.

I asked what her grandmother recognized in her and most appreciated about her. She said 'that I am lovable' and explained that being lovable meant many things. She listed them: she was a good person; she was warm; she was fun; she was normal; she was healthy; she was playful; she was receptive; she recognized good things in others.

Then, we spent a long time talking about how her life might have been different if she had lived with her grandmother. We developed the story of those differences through time, starting with when she was very little and coming all the way up to how things might be different for her now if she had grown up living with her grandmother.

I asked her to list again what her grandmother knew about her and wondered what life would be like if she owned those qualities about herself. She was more thoughtful than verbal in response to this last question.

Commentary

In response to a threatened re-emergence of the narrative of self-doubt and distress, Jessica is invited to search for previous life experience that contributes to knowledge of herself as 'healthy', 'normal', and 'playful'. Any memory of such experience will constitute an opening for story development around these ways of being.

In her search, Jessica discovers a real jewel. She is invited to relive the incident with her grandmother and examine its implications more closely. She accepts the invitation and makes the incident a more real, vivid, and meaningful part of her life narrative. She is then invited to experience the story from her grandmother's point of view. When she does, she gets a new view of herself. She can experience firsthand her grandmother's knowledge of her. This type of story development – incorporating other people's views – can be quite useful and effective.

Jessica is invited to construct and experience an alternative narrative about her whole life. To the extent that she becomes experientially involved in the world of this alternative story, the knowledge that she gains there will be available in this world as well. As we shall see later, the experience of this alternative story is a pivotal event in the therapy.

A further invitation is offered for Jessica to review and incorporate her grandmother's knowledge of her into her current life narrative. She responds by looking thoughtful, but not saying much.

The first phone call

Jessica called me five days after the fourth session. She began the conversation by asking, 'Do you know what it would be like to wear new shoes, new clothes, new makeup, and new breast implants all at the same time?' This was completely outside of my experience, so I asked her to explain. She told me that on the morning after our session, she drove through McDonald's on her way to work, as she had every morning, to pick up a cup of coffee. She was handed the coffee through her car window, as she had been every morning, and was asked if she would like sugar and cream, as she had been every morning, and automatically said, 'No, thank you' (not just, 'No', as she had every other morning). She found this quite startling and absolutely normal, at the same time.

She said now that she realized who she was, she knew that she was the kind of person who would say 'thank you', and so she did. Hearing herself actually say 'thank you' out loud was a startling and clear confirmation of her new identity. She did not remember ever having felt this strong for this many days in a row. She noticed that she was both more concerned about other people and more tuned in to herself. This was scary, too, because of how different it was. She was feeling strong all the time, but was afraid she must be denying other feelings because she couldn't believe she was so strong. She was afraid the changes were not real, and said that may have been why she used those unreal examples-breast implants and so on. But then she said, 'The neatest thing about this is I have something to guide me – my new image'.

Since the last appointment, she had also stopped smoking; this was because she now knew she was the kind of person who would not smoke. She said two things about stopping smoking that were particularly interesting to me, One was, 'Cigarettes are taking my energy and I need it for other things'. The other was that, in the past, when she was around people she liked, if they smoked, she smoked. She said that now it was important to be able to stay on her own path and have others go on their own.

She ended the phone call, saying, 'Having a new image of myself has affected me in ways I could never imagine. My car broke down, and I didn't meet the man of my dreams, but it's all right.'

Commentary

This whole conversation shows how experience of an alternative life narrative can bring forth changes in self-image, beliefs, and behavior. Most of the therapist's energy at times like this is expended in keeping up with all the changes.

The life narrative that was enriched so much in the previous session continues to make gains over the old, less pleasing one. These are changes that one could not have planned or predicted. One of the great joys of working in a narrative mode is witnessing the emergence of the rich and wonderful stories that people author for themselves.

The second phone call

Jessica called again eight days later. She had ended the relationship with her friend because she could not tolerate all the blaming. With everyone else, she reported, she was being her new self and liking it. When she was her new self with her friend, it began to seem like their relationship would end, so she would go back to her 'old' self. She now decided that she could not do that anymore, so she had ended the friendship. She felt strong but very sad. She believed that she was mourning the loss not only of her friend but of her old self.

I mused out loud about whether it was possible that the new self had been there all along, hidden under the effects of the abuse. That made sense to Jessica, but she said she was still sad. I said that I was not trying to take the sadness away. I was sad, too, that she had been through all that abuse and had been forced into hiding.

I asked about ways other than the sadness that her experience was different. She answered that she felt safer, more open, and more understanding. She said that this process had worked to give permission to parts of her that had already changed and to those ready and waiting to change, as well as giving her something she could use to live by every day, a new image of herself.

Commentary

As the new story expands and becomes dominant, the narrative of abuse and the effects of that narrative do not completely disappear; they just become less and less dominant. Jessica will probably always be able to access memories of the abuse and of how the effects of the abuse limited her life. However, those memories will be a much smaller part of her whole life narrative. In a complementary way, the 'new' story has always been with her.

Her sadness is accepted and affirmed. The subsequent question, about ways other than sadness that Jessica's experience is different, presupposes that as the new story continues to develop her experience of the world is different, and this invites her to story the differences. In so doing, she affirms that a new self-image goes hand-in-hand with her new story.

The fifth session

The fifth session was one month after the fourth. Jessica's very positive experience of getting to know herself in new ways had been interrupted and then overcome by a flood of graphic memories of the abuse that she had suffered. The central memory was of her uncle repeatedly thrusting his penis into her mouth while her father looked on. Her voice became very small and shaky as she described this memory. She reported that after it happened she went into the bathroom and washed out her mouth and then rode off on her bicycle.

I was very distressed to hear of this event. I looked directly at Jessica and said, 'I'm sorry that happened to you'.

Then, with her permission, I read her the notes from our two phone calls after the last session. She seemed to relax and began nodding as I read the notes. I said, 'You were telling me in that first phone call that you know the kind of person that you are. If you really owned that new self-image, and looked back through time with the knowledge and feelings that are part of the new self-image, what would you appreciate about the you that went through the abuse?'

'Appreciate?' she asked.

'Yeah, what can you appreciate or learn about the you that survived this abuse?'

As she reviewed the memories, Jessica identified that she was strong and resilient, and after some thought she even realized that she was creative. She silently began to weep. She said that, in the past, when she had these kinds of memories she had felt helplessness, terror, worthlessness, and shame, but she believed that this was the first time she had ever felt grief about everything she had endured. The grief felt like a good, pure feeling, signifying that she was worthy of sadness over something that had happened to her. We agreed that it was a joyful grief.

Commentary

The flood of images from the past is heard and accepted. Telling these gruesome tales from the past to a person in the present, who hears them as stories of the effects of the abuse and clearly separates her bad feelings about the abuse from her good feelings toward Jessica, tends to deconstruct their more horrifying aspects. No effort is made to develop them into more detailed stories. Instead, as Jessica is affirmed and accepted, she is invited to turn her attention back to the new story about herself that she has recently been developing and experiencing.

As Jessica begins to situate herself in the new story, she can experience herself as smart, tough, warm, tender, experienced, and so forth. Only as she shows evidence of 'owning' this new identity with its attendant characteristics is she invited to turn her attention back to the memories of abuse, and even then only in a specially structured way.

If she accepts the invitation, she is to 'look back through time' and look specifically for things to appreciate about her younger self. Previously, these memories had coached a story of helplessness, terror, worthlessness, and shame.

By connecting the memory with the preferred story and asking what she can appreciate about her younger self, Jessica is asked to restory the memories into ones of her capacity to survive and her positive identity. When Jessica looks back at her younger self through the eyes of her present self, she is able to appreciate that her younger self was strong, resilient, and creative in dealing with the effects of the abuse. This sets the stage for 'joyful grief'.

The third phone call

Three weeks later, Jessica called and said that she was thinking about canceling her next appointment. Her life was not perfect but she was feeling free. Her new image was guiding her, and the power had gone from the memories. Also, her car had broken down on the way home from the last appointment, and she had had to spend the night in a hotel. When things had been really bad, the three-hour drive each way seemed worth it, but now that things were going more smoothly for her, six hours seemed a long time to drive. She canceled the appointment, arranging to talk again a month later.

It seems from this report that Jessica is now rather solidly situating herself in a life narrative that supports a freer, more resourceful past, present, and future self-concept.

The fourth phone call

Jessica called again a month later. She said that before she had seen me she felt stuck, but now she was 'over the hump'. She liked herself. She was thinking about going back to her previous therapist for support in the new way she was thinking about herself and about life.

I asked her what had been most important in getting over the hump. She said it was the memory of singing with her grandmother and learning what her grandmother must have felt about her. It completely changed how she knew herself. I congratulated her on knowing herself and said I was curious to hear where her new knowledge might lead her. She thanked me, and we ended therapy.[7]

Commentary

As she wraps things up, Jessica affirms that the memory of singing with her grandmother was an opening that, when storied, helped her to revise her entire life narrative.

Jessica came to see me once more, four years later. We thought of ending our clinical example here, without including the later session, but on further reflection, we decided to include the rest of Jessica's story as we know it without explanatory comments, to show how far she was able to go in rescuing her romantic life from the effects of abuse. It also seems appropriate for her to have the last word about her therapy. It was particularly helpful to me that Jessica returned years later because her description of her life at the later time let me know that the re-authoring had really occurred in an enduring way and that she was living the future she had predicted for herself in earlier sessions.

The sixth session

Four years (to the day) after our last meeting, Jessica came to see me again. The first thing she told me was that she was buying a new house. I asked her what meaning this had for her. She said that it meant that she was going for what she wants and breaking family traditions.

She came to consult with me because she was involved, for the first time, in a romantic relationship. Gary, she told me, was different from her family. He was fun-loving, a traveler. He did not have traditional values about relationships between men and women. He was sexual and playful and did not use sex as power.

'If this works', Jessica said, 'I will be different from the women in my family'. I wondered if there was not a lot of evidence that she already was. She agreed that she was, but said that what worried her was that she reacted to Gary sexually like her sister and mother would. In her family she had learned that women are not supposed to like sex, and now she was finding intercourse painful. She reported that she was businesslike and efficient, wanting 'to get in, have an orgasm, and get out'.

When I asked how she was different from other people in her family, she said that she was the most playful person in her family. She had always had fun at school and work, but in recent years she has also played in other situations. She had taken up a number of team sports and thought that she had more fun in general than she used to. She also had more friends.

These changes led her to see herself as being more active, involved, and free. She listed friends who had noticed the changes and told me that some of her friends predicted that she would become involved with a man.

The preparation she had undertaken for these changes included coming to therapy and taking chances. For instance, she began frequenting a riding stable where she initially knew no one and joined a dart club as its only female member. She discovered that a lot of what is involved in play is being open to whatever pops into your mind. As she said this, she realized that there were precursors in her youth to these events. As a kid, she made something out of nothing and enjoyed daydreams. As a teenager, she got into telling jokes.

I summarized these events chronologically and asked what might come next. Jessica thought becoming more playful sexually and playing without structure would be next, but fear stood in the way of taking the next step and had also kept her from getting very close to Gary.

I wondered if going to a riding stable where she knew no one was an example of her overcoming fear. She agreed it was and added that she had become close friends with a man she met there. Other examples she offered of overcoming fear included being the only woman to join her dart club and telling Gary about her history of being abused and her subsequent difficulties.

I asked Jessica how she was able to overcome fear in these instances. She said that in the case of telling Gary about her history, she knew that because of the trouble she had with intimacy she would lose him if she did not tell him. So she took the risk and stood up to her own fearful internal dialogue. In a larger sense, Jessica said that she knew that a lot of what we fear in this world does not matter that much; she trusted her Higher Power and that helped her overcome fear.

I asked what these examples of taking risks and overcoming fear said about her. Jessica responded, 'that I can do it, that there is some part inside of me that is compelled to do it. I guess, also, that I have perseverance and a belief in my own growth and development.'

When I asked what difference it would make if she owned these descriptions of herself in the context of her relationship with Gary, she said that owning them could make a difference sexually. She grinned and said, 'It makes me want to practice more'. She added that she had been trying to please Gary, but this conversation was making her interested in practicing, like she had horseback riding and darts, for fun and so that she could relax. She also said that thinking about it as practicing made her feel like she could be more in charge. She intended to talk to Gary about these ideas.

As the session drew to an end, I asked Jessica if it had been helpful. She said, 'Yes. It hadn't occurred to me how much I have changed and accomplished until now'.

The fifth phone call

Jessica called one month later. After our session, she had talked with Gary about wanting to practice and be more in charge. They went through some 'misunderstandings about this but then things got comfortable'. Sex stopped hurting, and Jessica had been enjoying it more and more. She said that it got more playful and sensual. She and Gary had been having other problems, and she did not know if the two of them would end up together, but she felt very pleased with the possibilities she had begun to realize for herself as a sexual and playful person. She hoped the two of them would work things out but, if they did not, she understood that it was not because there was something wrong with her. It was because they did not 'fit'. She now believed that it was possible for her to have a satisfying intimate relationship.

Closing thoughts

We hope that the story of Jessica's therapy illustrates how narrative intentions guide our work and how the people we work with are the privileged authors of their own narratives. We feel privileged to be in on new narratives as they emerge and inspired by the new lives and relationships people author for themselves.

Acknowledgments

We would like to thank Froma Walsh for her careful reading and suggestions for revisions of an earlier draft of this chapter.

Notes

1. This chapter was originally published in M.F. Hoyt (ed) 1994: *Constructive Therapies*. New York: The Guilford Press.
2. The reference is not to this book, but to *Constructive Therapies*, in which this paper was first published.
3. Many people's ideas inform our work. We want to clearly acknowledge Michael White as being especially important in shaping our ideas and practices. We want to note that many people currently use a narrative metaphor with intentions and related actions that differ from ours. We are not trying here to represent the full range of narrative intentions, only to acquaint the reader with how the narrative metaphor shapes our current work.
4. You might want to try this yourself. Identify a behavior, perception, your recent life experience. Ask yourself how that behavior, experience, or emotion came about. Isn't you answer a story of sorts?
5. In many ways I felt that this therapy was really co-therapy. Jessica saw another therapist both before and after our work together. Much of the work we did was built on and later supported by work she did with the other therapist.
6. We prefer to start therapy, when possible, by learning some things about everyday, non-problematic roles, activities, and interests. As Dickerson and Zimmerman (1993) point out, it is important to begin by getting to know people as separate from problems and as experts on their own lives.
7. A colleague told us she would have been uneasy ending the therapy suddenly by phone. She wondered if the car breakdown evoked old terrors, or if fear blocked Jessica from getting closer to me. I did not have these thoughts. To me, it seemed that Jessica had entered a new narrative about herself and her life. Her therapy seemed successful. She did want support, but she knew that she needn't drive three hours each way to get it. Her ending therapy seemed a confirmation of her achievements.

10

Relationships and ethics:
Remembering what matters[1]

This paper was originally given as a keynote address. We have left the writing style in the form of a presentation, as if it was being delivered 'live' to people at a conference.

We don't know if this is true in Australia, but in North America every professional mental health association – the American Association for Marriage and Family Therapy, the National Association of Social Workers, the American Psychological Association, the American Psychiatric Association, just to name some – has a newsletter. And each of these newsletters has what's called an ethics column. Do you know what is the sole content of every one of those columns? A list of who is being kicked out of the organization and the rules they broke to get kicked out. When we first realized that the ethics columns of organizations we belong to consist of such thin and negative accounts, we were astounded. We began looking in other professional newsletters to find something that made more sense. There was nothing to be found. As many times as we have seen these columns, they continue to disturb us. We think differently about ethics. Our idea of an ethics report is not a list of who has been excluded from an organization.

As our experience with ethics columns so vividly showed us, the dominant culture of professional organizations favors ethics based on rules. To us, relational ethics make more sense. While rule-based ethics are universal and absolute, relational ethics are not. Relational ethics have to do with considering the effects of particular actions in particular contexts.

All ethics are based on discourses. For example, rule-based ethics concerning confidentiality have arisen within pathologizing discourses. If we think of problems as being located inside of people, if one of the first steps in facilitating change is to assign a pathological label, then complete privacy and confidentiality are fitting. The trouble is that as discourses change, ethical rules do not, because within the dominant culture those rules tend to be thought of as absolute, rather than as derived from discourses. So, even though, as narrative therapists, we challenge pathologizing discourses, maintaining that problems are not located in people, our professional organizations hold us accountable to rules of confidentiality. (We are not saying confidentiality is a bad thing. We do think, though, and our experience confirms, that outsider witness groups and other ways of being public can be very ethical practices for particular people, and there is little room for them within rules that emphasize confidentiality.)

What really disturbs us about rule-based ethics is that they stifle ethical thinking. They invite us *not* to think, not to consider the effects of a particular practice on a particular person or family, but simply to follow a rule. If we can avoid punishment, if we haven't been banished from a professional organization, we can assume that what we're doing is OK. It's as if we are either completely ethical or completely not ethical, rather than that we are human beings struggling with ethical dilemmas. When we try to talk about the difficulties we have with simply following rules, other therapists almost always ask, 'Are you saying anything goes?' and 'What about abuse?' There seems to be a very prevalent idea that if we are not following rules something calamitous will happen.

For us, it has been very much the opposite. When we followed ethical rules at times we did things that felt wrong. I (JF) once said 'No', I couldn't accept a ride home from the agency with a young person I was seeing in therapy who had recently bought his very first car. I now wonder if this rejection could have had more impact in a negative direction than the positive impact of all the work we did together. Recently, a colleague who was seeing a young person in therapy who was struggling with drug misuse phoned me (JF). The young woman had run away and my colleague had spoken to her parents, who were frantic, imagining their daughter strung out on drugs and vulnerable to all kinds of danger. I was seeing her best friend in therapy, which was something they had each talked freely about. My colleague called me and said, 'I'm going to ask you to do something totally unethical. Can you talk to your client about my client and ask her to pass along her parents' concerns to their daughter if she knows where her friend is? Maybe she could send back a message that would reassure them about her safety.' What struck me in that communication was his characterization of his request as being totally unethical. In terms of rules governing boundaries and confidentiality, yes. In terms of the effects of a friend being able to make a difference by passing along the concerns of her friend's parents, I don't think so.

Before we begin to describe some specific ways that we have put relational ethics into practice, we would like to quote Sue Jackson. In considering self-forgiveness Sue writes, 'I don't know about you, but I have done some bad things in my life. I have made mistakes that have had grave impacts on those I love. But it feels to me that, particularly in mid-life, the challenge is to come to terms with these omissions or commissions...' (2002 p.33). Similarly, we don't know about you, but we know we have done some bad things in our lives. We have made mistakes that have had grave impacts. Our purpose here is not to claim sterling ethical characters but to describe the impact of narrative ideas and practices in our personal and professional lives, particularly in terms of ethics and what matters.

In regard to mistakes and 'bad things', as Sue Jackson calls them, accountability practices, such as those developed by the Just Therapy Team at The Family Centre of Lower Hutt, New Zealand (Tamasese & Waldegrave 1994, Tamasese, Waldegrave, Tuhaka & Campbell 1998) have been transformative in our work and lives . Christopher McLean, Maggie Carey and Cheryl White have described how accountability practices:

> *... start from the recognition of the centrality of structured power differences in our society, and develop means of addressing them, so that groups that have been marginalized and oppressed can have their voices heard ... accountability ... is primarily concerned with addressing injustice. It provides members of the dominant group with the information necessary for them to stand against the oppressive practices implicit within their own culture, of which they will often be totally unaware.* (1996, p.5)

Accountability practices, as we have described them so far, were developed to help groups of people be accountable to each other – with emphasis on those in the more privileged group holding themselves accountable to those in marginalized groups. In our day-to-day practice as therapists with individuals, couples, and families, we are interested in being accountable on a person-to-person basis as well.

Rob Hall (1996) has pointed out how the accountability practices of which we speak are different than the practices associated with the top-down, rule-based accountability of patriarchal hierarchies. He calls the kind of accountability that we favor 'partnership accountability', emphasizing that goodwill, a commitment to constructing ethical solutions that promote social justice, critical self-appraisal, and responsibility, are necessary components of partnership accountability.

We'd like to tell you about two particularly meaningful experiences that, for us, have to do with accountability. And we'd like to tell them in a particular spirit. Five or six years ago I (JF) was at a very large conference. There was a banquet for lunch. Hundreds of us were seated at round tables of 12, pushed close together, filling a ballroom. There was a lull in the conversation at my table and I could clearly hear a woman talking at an adjoining table, seated back-to-back with me. She was talking about supervision, and I quickly realized that she was talking about a two-year program she had recently completed at our center. She was recounting her experience of doing therapy with a reflecting team. 'I had been in a different family therapy training program before', she said. 'I dreaded my turn to do therapy. All eyes were on me. It felt like they were judging my work and I was acutely aware of every wrong move. But with a reflecting team', she said. 'it was completely different. I had the feeling of the whole team supporting me. I knew that if I didn't notice something important, someone on the team would weave it into the conversation. It wasn't about judging. We were all in it together. It was about learning how to do the work.'

We offer these stories in a similar spirit. We'd like to think of you as our team during this plenary, and that way we can tell some meaningful stories that might be difficult to tell otherwise.

Working with Margaret

The first story we are going to tell concerns my (GC) work as a therapist and my attempts to be accountable to a woman named Margaret. I really made a serious mistake with Margaret. In other settings, governed by other discourses, I might well feel so much shame and fear so much censure about my mistake that I wouldn't choose to tell this story. However, in this setting, I know there are friends and colleagues who will serve as a supportive outsider witness group while I acknowledge the mistake and practice accountability for it – a process that need not involve shame or censure.

I saw Margaret and her family twice; the first time with Jill and the second time, because of scheduling difficulties, by myself. Before we met, Margaret and her partner, Steven, had decided to divorce. However, when they came to therapy, they all still lived together – against Margaret's wishes. Margaret described being upset by Steven's angry and domineering actions, especially those he directed at their 14-year-old daughter, Claire. Steven had shoved Claire into walls and spat on her. He continually threatened her with bodily harm, and at the time we met he was cursing at her and saying disrespectful and demeaning things on a daily basis. The authorities had been made aware of the situation, but deemed that even though Margaret experienced these actions as terrifying, they were not severe enough to warrant intervention. Except during explosive confrontations, Claire was not speaking to Steven at all. Margaret was worried about how things should be handled while Steven was still in the house and thought that therapy could provide a forum for planning the transitional time.

Steven said that Claire and Margaret were exaggerating, and he wanted to maintain the best relationship he could with his children. Claire (the elder daughter) said that she did not want to be involved in anything having to do with Steven. Erin, the 7-year-old, said that she wanted the family to stay together.

At the second meeting, which we had previously agreed was to focus on Claire's and Steven's relationship, Margaret said that Steven had been emotionally and physically abusive to Claire. When I began to question Claire, she answered in monosyllables and then, announcing that she did not want to be involved, walked out.

After Claire left, Steven said firmly, 'There is nothing to talk about'.

I attempted to address whether Margaret and Steven felt that Steven could continue to be in the house and whether Claire would be safe. Margaret said she did think some of the things Steven said to Claire were very damaging, but that Claire was keeping the interactions to a minimum. Steven seemed very resentful and unwilling to speak to me in any full way. He said he did not think family therapy was appropriate for a family that had already decided to break up.

Margaret suggested that family therapy might help *how* they broke up and might improve their relationships for the rest of their lives. Steven said that he had participated in enough family therapy and that everything had already been said. (He was referring to a number of therapies the family had participated in prior to the decision to divorce.)

We have since learned that Margaret's experience and mine were quite different from this point on. I can now see how my stance and words in the interview obscured Margaret's voice, so it is no surprise that I did not hear her thoughts during the session. As you will learn soon, even though she experienced no room in the interview, Margaret did not break off the relationship with me. It is her persistence, not my sensitivity or skill, that makes it possible for us to report both experiences – hers and mine – to you. We will present Margaret's and my thoughts as a kind of dialogue:

GC: It seemed to me that Steven had made up his mind not to participate further in family therapy.

M: I knew that Steven would try to run away from any attempt to confront his abuse. I prayed that this time I would have help in sustaining the confrontation, for my daughter's sake.

GC: I thought that family therapy would either be superficial and rather meaningless or would be yet another arena for the violence and abuse. It would be easier and safer for everyone to keep their distance and pursue the divorce.

M: Steven delayed the divorce at every turn, and he continued to live in the same house, against my wishes, treating Claire in the same violent and abusive ways, for two more years.

GC: I knew that Steven, Claire, and Margaret were all in individual therapy. I hoped that they would be able to address the impact of these problems more freely in those settings.

M: After years of couple and individual therapy, Steven's abuse at home was, if anything, escalating. He quoted his individual therapist in support of his abusive conduct, saying that she had told him that his daughter was unusually difficult, and that it was therefore understandable that he lost his temper. Claire generally could not trust or connect with any individual therapist she had seen enough to discuss the abuse she was enduring at home. The one time Claire tried to bring the issue up with her individual therapist, Steven went to talk with the therapist, and Claire's therapist had then refused to take the abuse seriously.

GC: Although Margaret was interested in family therapy, it seemed that at that point no one else in the family was. I said that it wasn't possible to force someone to talk, and perhaps since they were separating, the individual therapies could provide individual help and support.

M: Here I am, alone again in trying to voice and face what's wrong in this family. Maybe I'm imagining it, maybe things aren't so bad, maybe it's just me. I guess I was crazy to try this, what a stupid idea.

A week after the second interview, Margaret's therapist called to tell me about Margaret's disappointment and discouragement over what had happened in the family meeting. Margaret felt that I had sided with Steven. I told the therapist that it must have felt like there was a lot of male energy in the room. I wondered how things might have been different if Jill had been there. The therapist reported our conversation back to Margaret.

It was not Margaret's responsibility to let me in on her experience beyond this point, but she did. She wrote me a three-page letter in which she carefully described how I had shut down the communication process and supported Steven's avoidance. She made it clear how she believed it was vital that there be some witnessing of the abuse that had occurred in their family. She brought to life for me how the session had invalidated her goals and left her feeling crazy and shut down.

I am grateful that she did this. I am grateful that she held me accountable by speaking to her therapist, that her therapist called me, and that Margaret wrote her letter.

Nevertheless, when I got the letter I was mortified. Distressed and shaken, I consulted Jill so I could hear how a woman might have experienced the situation differently, and how that different experience might have led to different behavior.

Jill thought I had approached the meeting more oriented to action than she would have been. When I could not see a way to make something happen, I gave up. She wondered what it would have been like to ask more questions and listen more patiently – with my heart as well as my ears. She suggested I consult Margaret about what I had missed in her experience: her hopes, her fears, and her understandable anger at not being heard.

I thought that was a really good idea, but I wasn't sure whether Margaret would be willing to meet with me again for any purpose. In further conversation with Jill, I decided to contact Margaret and ask if she would be willing to consult with me so that I might apologize face-to-face, and so that I might learn how to be more useful to women in circumstances similar to hers in the future. As I would be benefiting from her experience and knowledge, I said that I would pay her at my hourly clinical rate for any time she was willing to give to this project. Margaret did agree to meet with me and serve as my consultant.

Hearing Margaret's reflections on the therapy, I was able to imagine things I could have said and done that might have honored her hopes that the abuse would be addressed; that she and Steven could work together to minimize its effects on the entire family. The things that Margaret helped me see have guided me in other situations where I have been called on to witness, name, and deal with abuse. I am thankful to Margaret for this, and I am also thankful that rules about professional boundaries didn't keep me from this experience.

If there had not been a clearly established tradition of partnership accountability practices in narrative therapy, Jill and I probably wouldn't have come up with this way of addressing the mistake I made. The second therapy interview could have remained a confirmation for Margaret that there was something wrong with her. Instead, she said that our response empowered her and helped heal the wound to her dignity. For me, the consultation was a turning point in the way I work with violence and abuse.

When we thought about writing about our experience with Margaret, I (JF) called her to find out what that would be like for her – not just to ask her permission, but to find out if it would feel like a good thing rather than exploitation. She actually was enthusiastic about this further project. I asked her to go over with me her experience of the consultation so that we would not privilege our experience over hers. I set up a time, and at that time I called her back to interview her about her memories of serving as Gene's consultant.

Margaret told me that she had hoped that Gene would call but had not been confident that he would. A previous male therapist had been willing to talk with her about problems and mistakes in therapy but had never taken responsibility for them. Gene questioned his role and thought about what had happened. Margaret said, 'It undid the feeling of being crazy in the session. It turned the world right side up again.' His comment that there was a lot of male energy in the room signaled Margaret that it was not a given for him that whatever happened had to do with her issues. It was that that encouraged her to take the time to write the letter.

I took careful notes of these and other things she said as we talked, then combined them with our recollections to construct a draft account of the whole incident.

We sent Margaret Jill's draft, and after she had time to review it, I (GC) met with her to refine our collaborative telling of the story. We again paid Margaret at my hourly clinical rate for helping and advising us. Also, we have committed to talking with her at any time about the ongoing effects on her life of this whole series of interactions.

Margaret has since come to see me a number of times to consult about other problems. I (GC) can't tell you what a surprise and delight the first call was. For me, the trust her continuing consultation shows is a vivid confirmation of the transformative nature of accountability practices.

Being Jewish in Germany

The groundwork for another experience having to do with partnership accountability began more than two years ago when I (JF) was teaching in Munich. I was very much enjoying the group and my experience there until I began to talk about the politics of the work. Suddenly a second set of thoughts became almost palpable, pulling me away from what I was presenting. 'Do you realize that you, a Jewish woman, are talking about politics in Germany?' they whispered urgently. 'What would your grandparents think?' I looked around at the group of Germans and Austrians joining together with me, responding from their hearts, intent on striving for social justice through their work, and I continued speaking about these matters of great importance to me.

When we broke for lunch, I walked with new friends, looking at old stone streets and house fronts. With each step I wondered, 'What happened here? And here? And right here?' And in my mind's eye I saw flashes of blood, looks of betrayal, panic, pain, stomping boots. I was overwhelmed, as though the people who had once lived there were beckoning me. I was afraid.

My host, Rudi Kronbichler, had become a trusted friend. He brought up the current politics in Austria with concern. He took clear stands and I knew I was safe talking with him. But I couldn't speak. 'Do you know I'm Jewish?' I wondered. 'Does everyone in the group?' 'How do I talk about fears from before my lifetime with someone who grew up in Austria and spoke to me in a second language?'

When the workshop was over I went to Salzburg. Alone in my hotel room I checked e-mail. A message from Stevie, my brother, flashed across my screen. I'm on his buddy list. I poured out my experience and was frightened to let him go. I felt a slender thread stretched across continents, connecting me to safety. When we finally said good-bye I sat on my bed and trembled.

I wrote about this experience (Freedman 1999) and then realized I had no choice but to talk to Rudi about it before he read the published version. We had a brief e-mail conversation about it and decided to talk in person several months later when he would be coming to Evanston for a workshop. When the time came, we sat in a Jewish deli in a suburb of Chicago and I told him about my experience. He listened quietly, nodded, looked me directly in the eye and said, 'When you come to Salzburg will you come with me to Mauthausen, the concentration camp?' I said 'Yes', immediately and he said, 'Are you sure, Jill? Think about it'.

I did think about it in the months before I returned to Salzburg, and it seemed like an important thing to do. This time, no frightening thoughts or voices interrupted my workshop in Salzburg. And no trembling alone in the hotel. The day after the workshop ended was the appointed day for our journey to Mauthausen. It stormed all the way there. How can I describe the feeling of walking up those stone steps and seeing the yard where the train journey ended and people lined up to face forced labor or gas chambers?

The concentration camp is now a well-preserved national monument. We began by watching a documentary detailing what happened there. As we heard the testimony of someone who had been the local delivery boy during Mauthausen's construction insist that the villagers knew what was happening there, the sorrow and grief I experienced from my first glimpse of the camp began to harden and include a sense of foreboding. As we heard reports of the atrocities that occurred in this place that took 200,000 lives, I felt an intense sense of horror and a heaviness that I had never before experienced. I felt weighed down to that very spot, unable to move, and frozen away from Rudi. I longed to share my anguish, yet felt unable to even look at Rudi, who somehow for me had stopped being a person I knew and had become instead a generic German (never mind that he is from Austria). I witnessed wooden bunks smaller than single beds that slept three like sardines. I saw gas chambers, ovens, and graveyards. I think I ceased to breathe, feeling so much and laboring to express nothing to this generic German I was stuck with. And then, we approached the 'Stairway of Death' the film had documented. The stairway led to a huge pit that camp inmates had labored in until they dropped. A witness told how Jews were forced to stand in line at the top of that pit and each was forced, at gunpoint, to push the person in front of him off the edge to certain death. I heard a sharp intake of breath and turned to look directly at Rudi for the first time in perhaps, an hour and a half. Tears were streaming down his face. And I felt my heart open. We held each other briefly and then I stood back and looked into the pain on his face. We reached for each other's hand and pledged out loud that we stood united and opposed to anything that would support that kind of hatred and atrocity ever happening again.

On the way home to Salzburg, we talked. I asked all the questions I had been afraid to ask and didn't even know I had been afraid to ask. The most important one for me was 'Do you feel responsible?' and I had just a small moment of fear that he would say it all happened before he was born. But he didn't. Unflinchingly, he said, 'Yes. I am responsible as an Austrian', and he went on to tell me what that was like and what his experience was as a child visiting Mauthausen and asking adults about the war and feeling the difficulty with which they answered.

Recently I was with some friends who are Jewish. Somehow the conversation led me to begin to talk about this experience. They were horrified and asked, 'Why would you want to do that?' It was then that I realized this experience, which was freeing and important, was supported by my immersion in a narrative worldview. I grew up with extended family and friends who were against buying anything German or in any way supporting anything German. I now understand how a view of internalized pathology makes this kind of totalizing judgment possible. It also freezes people in the worst possible circumstances. I have now experienced firsthand the healing power of accountability, which contributes to the world moving beyond stories of unfathomable horror.

To us, these are stories of ethics in action – the kind of ethics that look not to rules but to the effects of what we do. These are ethics that are not about kicking people out but about practicing a kind of accountability that opens up possibilities for bringing people together to address mistakes and wrongdoing. I don't think we are going too far when we suggest that these kinds of ethical acts contribute to making the world a better place.

Ethics in community

Engaging in these ethical practices is not something that we could do alone. We, of course, have each other. But we also have a larger community. We are lucky enough to have a community in our hometown – Evanston, Illinois, USA. But that is relatively new. What has sustained us in adopting this worldview, long before we were joined by others in Evanston, is a community of people in our hearts and minds who inspire us and with whom we feel joined. At times we talk with each other about what those people would do if they were facing a particular dilemma we are facing. At other times we have found the strength to carry through a particular action by feeling their solidarity of purpose with us. Some people have become members of our community through a fleeting, but important, one-time association. Others we will see again and again. Some have become members through our witnessing of their words or practices, rather than through a relationship with us. Through joining with these people in our hearts and minds we are more in touch with what we stand for. We've decided not to name names here, but I can't resist naming just one. I (JF) hold Rudi Kronbichler close as a member of my community, admiring him for inviting me to go with him to Mauthausen and openly sharing his experience with me.

We imagine that as we speak at least one person will come to mind for you … someone who has been a source of inspiration, whose actions or words you admire or who stands for what is most important to you. Perhaps this person could be a more closely held part of your community, even if you might never meet them again face-to-face.

We would like to invite you to take a few minutes to identify such a person (if you haven't already) and to reflect on how you might use your actual or virtual relationship with that person to lovingly critique your practices and to carry on when the going gets hard ... Would you be willing to do that? If you are, consider the following questions as we ask them:[2]

- How is this person important to you?
- What do you know more clearly and strongly about yourself or about the world when you are with this person? (Or if you imagine being joined with this person?)
- What values or purposes or aspirations does this person help you put into action?
- What difference might it make in your daily work if this person vividly accompanied you there in your heart and mind?

Summary

At this point we would like to summarize a few points that we hope have been implicit in our presentation so far.

- The ethics that we follow are relational ethics.
- Relational ethics lead us to reflect critically on the effects of our actions in particular contexts with particular people.

- To engage in a useful critique of our actions, we require a community of people who are joined with us around that purpose.
- The experience of carefully reflecting on and deconstructing the effects of our actions within a community of concern is quite different than the experience of being 'under the gaze' – that experience that can arise so easily under the scrutiny of hierarchical, rule-based ethics.
- In a community of shared purpose, we can find the willingness to be moved, to open our hearts to other peoples' particular dilemmas and struggles.
- In community, we can tell and retell the stories that people find meaningful, thus spreading the waves of meaning.
- As meaning spreads, its significance grows. For example, Margaret knows we are telling her story here in Canberra. She knows this might help others who are struggling with abuse, and that knowledge sustains her, helping her courage and confidence grow as the grip of the violence weakens.

Perhaps the thing that has most attracted and engaged us in this work that has come to be called narrative therapy is the way its practices and its ethics support and enrich each other. If we could convince you to stay and listen to us talk all day rather than attending your other workshops, we'd consider with you other narrative practices such as situating ourselves, reflecting practices, and documenting and circulating insider knowledges, that help keep us centered in relational, rather than rule-based ethics. Instead, we will conclude by sharing just one other story that has to do with ethics, relationship, and community.

Mary

This story began for me (JF) with the breaking of one of those absolute rules, the one about dual relationships. Mary is a psychologist who I had developed some closeness with as she attended several of our workshops. When she called me to initiate therapy she said that she knew she 'shouldn't' ask me because of our previous relationship but she didn't know anyone else who would take this important path with her. Mary's partner, Sy, had died just a few months earlier, in his mid-forties, of melanoma. In the first weeks and months Mary's family and friends were wonderfully supportive. But after a few months they began to talk with her about letting go and moving on. Mary was very clear that she didn't want to let go or move on. As she told me, 'Sy didn't want to go and we didn't want him to. There will be no letting go here.' But her friends who had offered unfailing support in the first months, began first to push and then to show disapproval. Mary told me that she wanted help in continuing the relationship with Sy. I agreed to join her. And entered one of the most meaningful therapeutic relationships that I've ever had.

When we were asked to speak about what matters, the work with Mary immediately came to mind. This relationship mattered to her and to me and to many others who have joined us through watching this tape. As we join the conversation, I've just been asking Mary what Sy most appreciated about her.

[transcript of video tape]

Jill: I just am wondering what the experience of the battle against cancer was like. What he saw in you? In your oneness with him around that battle against cancer ...

Mary: Wait, say that again?

J: I've just been thinking that there are so many different ways people respond to a scary diagnosis. And that he was with somebody who joined, and said, 'we, this is our battle'. And, I'm just wondering what that was like for him to have you be his partner in that battle? And to take the stance that you took ... I think that that made the whole experience of going through that a different one; a very different one.

M: Oh, yeah. I think I made it very intimate.

J: And I guess I'm wondering what he must have appreciated in your being right there with him through that.

M: I think that I was right there with him through that. Yeah. I think he appreciated that.

J: Mmm hmm.

M: All the way through to the very end. To the last breath. I was with him.

J: And what did he know about you? And your willingness to do that?

M: He would say I was committed. That I loved him. And that … well, that love is more powerful than fear.

J: Mmm hmm.

M: That love is more powerful than fear. And he taught me to claim that in myself.

J: I was just wondering if it changed your relationship with yourself to have that kind of relationship with him?

M: It really has. It's also changed my relationship with my friends.

J: How?

M: Well, I realize that love is more powerful than fear. I mean, in a strange way, the night he died was just like the night we met. A beginning and an end kind of thing.

J: Huh huh.

M: The night that we met, he was a graduate student in the department next to me. And a *blabber*! Just like our youngest son, who we call the announcer. He loved to talk. And he was so fascinating. He had big stories and I loved it. I was having this dilemma about something, at the time, I forget what, but we started talking. We started talking at like one o'clock, and then it got to be like five o'clock, maybe. And he said, 'Well, do you want to go out for a pizza?' And I said, 'Well, yeah, great'. It was a Friday night, so we went to the Pizza Inn and just sat there. I sure don't remember the pizza, but we sat there until it closed, just talking.

J: Mmm.

M: And I remember thinking, wow, a guy could be this kind of a friend. We could have sat all night long talking. And I just loved it. The night he died was sort of the same way, you know? We told stories all night long. It took me a while to put love in front of fear. It took some time. I had to sit back and just pray. I said the Serenity Prayer about eighty times and he was laughing while I was doing it. I was at the side of his bed, just saying it out loud. And he was laughing. Every time I said it, he would laugh. And, every time I said it I would throw in another stupid option, like, 'Go to the phone and call your best friend' or 'Go down the hall and check with the nurse'.

J: Mmm hmm.

M: And then, all of a sudden, I knew what to do. Just tell him all the wonderful stories of your life together! All the best stories. And I started at the beginning. In sort of the way we're doing now. And I just started telling him stories. And he was laughing. And between stories he would do his management stuff. Like, he would say to me, 'Don't forget. Get forty copies of the death certificate.'

J: (Laughs)

M: And, I was like, 'Jeez!' It's like, 'Right now you are dying, and you are taking care of us!' You know?

J: Yeah.

M: It gave me the courage to just, beam more love. And it gave him the courage, I think, to beam more love at me.

J: Mmm hmm.

M: And he would say things like, 'Mary, all of the unpaid bills are on the right hand side of the desk. Don't forget! And the insurance ... you can find that in the second folder.' So, I think as my telling the love stories got stronger, he kept coming back with extra stuff I'd need. (Mary laughs warmly)

J: (Joins in the laughter)

M: It was so *something*, you know? And, he was smiling through these stories. And I would tell him more love stories, you know. And he'd go, 'Yeah, yeah, yeah'. Right up until ... all of a sudden he had this stroke. His eyes went back ... And then he started to breathe this very deep breathing ... And I got right up on his face. And I just held on to him. And I thought, 'As long as you can breathe, I can say I love you'. So ... He would breathe ... And I would say, 'I love you'. And then he would breathe and I would say, 'I love you'. And then he stopped breathing.

Just before – maybe two minutes before he stopped breathing – his doctor came in, who was a sweetheart, a *sweetheart*! And I didn't even care. I said, 'Just leave me alone'. And I just kept right on being with Sy. And then Sy took his last breath.

The doctor leaned over and kissed him right on the head. And he said, 'There was a man!' And I know that doctor doesn't kiss everybody on the head. (Mary is laughing and crying at the same time.)

J: (Jill is too.)

M: I had been frightened ... But, it was sort of like love really didn't make it fearful. It was just like, 'How can I make this going away from me the best? Because I love you.' (Crying freely) Love is a powerful thing. You should only marry people you love. (Laughs with the tears)

J: (Is joined with Mary in the laughter and tears)

M: So, I like this idea of seeing myself – my creative points – through his eyes. I think it would give me more courage.

J: I can't imagine more courage, Mary.

M: Well, I can.

J: Well maybe I can learn something about that from you.

The usual discourse in our culture about loss and grief is to let go and move on. Mary knew that that was not what she wanted to do but she was losing her entire support system as she stood up to that set of ideas. In many ways, the entire therapy was simply creating a context in which it was OK not to live out the prevailing discourse, but to work instead on ways that Sy could continue to live on in the life of Mary and their children and that Mary and Sy's relationship could continue. This continuing of relationship is an idea that is very much a part of some cultures, but not of Mary's.

This left Mary in a position of needing to invent ways to continue the relationship. One thing that she did was set up an easel in the family room where she painted a portrait of Sy during the time that I saw her in therapy. At first her children were horrified by her project and asked her at least to move it out of their primary living space. She refused. This portrait of Sy is made up entirely of the names of those he loved and those who loved him. Mary's name forms his lips, his children's form his eyes, his sister is waves through his hair. As Mary painted, her children began watching and then began making suggestions for where the name of a friend or neighbor might be included.

Mary's portrait brings us again to the importance of community. We made the tape at Mary's request because she wanted a record of this time to share with her children, but it didn't stop there. She has been happy for us to show this tape in settings like this because she hopes it will support others in standing up to the discourse of letting go and moving on. We've shown this tape around the world and sometimes people have been moved to respond. To complete this presentation. we'd like to read you some letters that Mary received from some therapists in Christchurch, New Zealand, who saw this tape at a workshop we did there about a year ago..

Dear Mary,

I have participated in the sharing of your experience of your husband's death by viewing a video. Now I am sitting on a grassy riverbank in Christchurch writing to you. A plane is flying noisily overhead and the cicadas are noisy in the summer trees. I am deeply touched by your experience, in fact stunned. When you spoke of the joy of being able to share that last night telling stories and the intimacy of being so close and together I could understand what you meant and am so glad for you that you have such a beautiful memory of love to keep in your spirit.

Dear Mary,

I have just had the privilege of viewing a videotape of a therapy session you did with Jill, which she showed as part of a workshop she and Gene have just run here in Christchurch. I was very moved by it. I am English born and we are not known for our depth of feeling – unless it's to do with football – but listening to your responses and watching your animation when you spoke of your husband Sy and of how you see yourself through his eyes led me to wonder how I might talk differently with my brother, John, who lost his only son Callum two years ago through suicide at only 21 years. I have another way of looking at Callum now and can look beyond the 'why?' I can also begin to see myself in a different light, to see myself the way Callum might have seen me – I was there on the day of his birth and again on the day of his death (to identify him for the police). But more, I feel for John. What I see is that he has succumbed very much to the cultural norm here, especially among 'kiwi blokes' which is to tuck it away, not talk about his son's death, get on with life, work, family. And he can't. Not really! So considering these new ideas has given me hope and encouragement that John and I may perhaps be able to have conversations about Callum in ways that are different than what he's experienced so far and which may open new windows on how he sees himself in relation to Callum. Thank you.

Dear Mary,

I wanted you to know how your tape touched my life. I work as a counsellor and in my work have re-membering conversations with people I see. But until today I have never asked myself what my first husband might have appreciated about what I brought to his life. He died of cancer 28 years ago when we were both 24. As I begin to think about that lots of stories are beginning to come into my mind. As it happens, tonight some very good friends are having a surprise 30th wedding anniversary party. He and I were part of the wedding party – me as a bridesmaid. He as best man. So I would have been thinking of him today but now I will be thinking differently.

Dear Mary,

Among my stories is the loss of my 8-month-old daughter Nina 25 years ago ... 3 years ago I visited Notre Dame. I had been asked by a friend to light a candle for her mother. I found myself in a quiet alcove in front of a bare stand. I collected a candle and thought of my friend. And that reflection led me to light candles for Nina and others. I remember standing in front of the stand, all spaces filled with lit candles and as I allowed myself to embrace that sense of loss, I had a sense of all those people before me who had stood at this stand doing as I had done and of all those people who will come after me. And felt joined, embraced, part of the huge humanness of it all. It was such a powerful feeling. Today watching and listening to your story I felt that joining again and I thank you for the specialness, the integrity, the joy, and the sadness. Love is more powerful than fear.

Thank you.

Notes

1. This paper was presented as a keynote address at the 4th Australian Narrative Therapy and Community Work Conference held in Canberra in April 2002.
2. At this point in the presentation we invited the audience members to consider their responses to these questions, and gave them the following instructions: 'When you are ready, turn to someone beside you and introduce them to this person you have decided to include more closely in your community. You might want to tell them how you know this person or perhaps a story about them or about your relationship with them. Take about 3 minutes each way to introduce this member of your community.'

   After these three minutes had passed we then said, 'Now, consider how holding this person more closely in your heart and mind will make a difference in confronting difficult dilemmas or reflecting on aspects of your work that might be problematic. Consider how this person's presence might help you in practicing accountability. Take a couple of minutes to talk with your neighbor about how holding this person close will make a difference.'

   After two minutes we then said, 'We have been talking about community and yet because of time constraints have limited this conversation to one person you would like to hold more closely. But we invite you as the conference goes on and after the conference is over to consider other people you'd like to hold close as members of your community.'

PART FOUR

Exercises

Finally, we have included here two exercises that we have developed for training contexts. In our experience, developing training exercises about narrative practice is one way to further clarify our understandings. The process of creating an exercise takes us to unexpected places and this is a real pleasure. To us, the experience of making an exercise can be similar to learning to play a difficult piece of music. There is a certain pleasure in engaging with something that requires our total focus. When people then take the exercises we've developed in their own unique directions it is very rewarding. We're really pleased to be able to include the following two exercises here, both of which document workshops that we have held at Dulwich Centre Publications' International Narrative Therapy and Community Work Conferences in Adelaide, South Australia.

11

Developing relationships, performing identities [1]

Since engaging with narrative ways of working, one of the aspects we have found most helpful is the idea that identity can be approached as a project. We make ourselves and each other up through the directions in life that we choose. Different possibilities for identity are opened through examining and revising relationships with problems and relationships with particular discourses and cultures. Equally significant possibilities are created by exploring ways of further developing thick and rich experiences of the relationships we have in our lives with other people.

When we think back on our workshop we remember the people who were there - the stories they told, the looks on their faces, how they made the room come alive. They joined with us in telling stories about and honouring the relationships in each of our lives that shape and sustain our preferred identities - our 'best selves'. Together we reflected on narrative practices, unpacking the many ways that they can bring forth new relational identities. We showed video-tapes of some of the people we work with talking about places and people who contributed to their identities, and we did an exercise to explore some of the ways narrative practices can be used in projects having to do with identity.

We put up the following lists on the overhead. We hope they give you a hint of some of the discussions we had, first about dominant discourses in our culture that stand in opposition to ideas of relational identity, and then about some of the narrative practices that build on and help develop the experience of relational identity.

Discourses that interfere with notions of relational identity

The following is a list of names that hint at different overlapping discourses, each of which is at odds with a relational experience of identity. It is not a complete list, and the names we use here may not be the ones that you would use. We would be curious to know what you experience as you read through the list. Are there important discourses that aren't mentioned here? If so, we would be interested in hearing your additions to the list.

- Separation/individuation
- 'Rugged individualism' (the loner-hero)
- Othering (dividing practices)
  - Individual, pathology-based diagnosis
  - Racism
  - Classism
  - Heterosexism
  - Nationalism
- Self
  - 'Essential' or 'core' self
  - Self-actualisation
  - Self-esteem
  - Self-reliance
  - Self-policing
- Person as container (container metaphors)
  - Inner strength
  - Self-contained
  - Resources (finding it within)
  - Inner child
  - Repression (of emotion, for example) and the need for expression

- Boundaries

  'Strong fences make good neighbours'

  Psychological discourses that privilege confidentiality, containment, and individuality over spreading the news, interdependence, and community

Narrative practices that presuppose the notion of relational identity

Some readers may not be familiar with all these practices; others may not see clearly how some practices presuppose and rely on the notion of relational identity. Nevertheless, we hope that reading over this list will give you some experience of how important relational notions of identity are to this work.

- Re-membering
- Documents (documenting new relationships with problems and projects)
- Letters
- Leagues/teams
- Outsider witness groups (reflecting teams)
- Accountability practices
- Situating
- Collaborating
- Externalising (changing relationships with problems)
- Inquiry into the effects of discourses (questioning relationships with discourses)
- 'Taking it back' practices
- De-centering

With these ideas in mind, we offered the following exercise as a way for people to explore some aspects of relational identity in their own lives, and, in so doing, perhaps to re-experience and thicken preferred aspects of their identities. We now offer this exercise to you. It is written to be done in pairs, but you could also guide yourself through it step by step.

Exercise: Relational identity

In pairs, ask your partner to identify:

- Someone from the past who she has always known was a significant person in her life.
- A group, ideology, or movement that she has felt very much a part of (for example, the anti-war movement, a church, or a sports team).
- A problem with which she has revised her relationship.

Then help your partner to develop three different sketches of herself as she knows herself through her relationships with the people or things identified above.

Start by asking your partner to tell the story of the relationship, and then ask questions that invite her to name her identities in the different relationships.

Sample questions for relationship 1:

- *Can you tell me a bit about your relationship with this person?*
- *What did this person most appreciate about you?*
- *If you saw yourself through this person's eyes, how would you describe yourself?*
- *What were you in touch with about yourself when you were with this person?*
- *What did your being this way (the way described in the answers to the above questions) contribute to this person's life?*
- *How would you describe your identity in this relationship?*

Sample questions for relationship 2:

- *Can you tell me about your participation in this group or movement?*
- *If you actively chose this group or movement, what about it attracted you?*
- *What were you affiliating with in joining this group or movement?*
- *What can you see in yourself in reviewing your participation?*
- *What did you contribute to this group or movement?*

- *If I could interview other members, what might they tell me about you? What was it like having a sense that others saw you in this way?*
- *How [these could be very small ways] was this group or local version of the movement different for your having participated in it?*
- *Were there times in relation to this group or movement when you felt like you were participating in something larger than yourself? What was that like?*
- *How would you describe your identity in this relationship?*

Sample questions for relationship 3:

- *Can you tell me about this problem as you used to experience it? What were some of this problem's effects back then?*
- *What has changed about your relationship with this problem? How did that change come about? Were other people important in facilitating this change?*
- *Now that you have changed your relationship with the problem, what is different about your life and relationships?*
- *What do you know now about yourself that you didn't know when the problem was obscuring your view?*
- *How does your new relationship with this problem affect your contributions in the world?*
- *If the problem could speak, what would it most respect about you as a 'worthy adversary'?*
- *How did changing your relationship with the problem change your identity?*
- *How would you name or describe your identity in this new relationship with the problem?*

Now, ask your partner to imagine, one at a time, seeing herself in each of these identities (or, if she already sees herself in this identity, ask her to see herself *more fully* in it). Here are some sample questions for this part:

- *Is each of these different than your usual view? How?*
- *Do you like seeing yourself in each of these ways? Why?*
- *What difference would it make in your life and ongoing affiliations to keep each of these views alive?*

- *What difference would it make to the communities in which you participate if you more fully embodied these things in your day-to-day life?*

Conclude this round by having a conversation about the process, the differences in the three views, and about whether there is a place (or could be a place) in your partner's life for all of them.

In conclusion, we'd like to say that this idea of relational identity has been a very enriching one for us, and one we've come to relatively late in life. That is, it is not part of the culture that either of us were raised in. We discovered at the conference that Aboriginal people have long had knowledge of relational identity. Our experiences in Italy lead us to believe that Italian people also value creating their identities through relationship. We feel fortunate to be able to share in some of these practices that for others have been ways of life for generations. We hope that the exercise enriches your experience of relational identity and inspires you to find new ways to make use of the experience in your life and work.

Note

1. This exercise was originally published in Dulwich Centre Publications 1999: *Narrative Therapy and Community Work: A conference collection. Adelaide: Dulwich Centre Publications*

12

Therapy relationships that open possibilities for us all:

The narratively informed therapeutic relationship[1]

This was an interactive workshop. Many of the ideas in this paper were suggested by participants. We apologise if in this written representation of the workshop we have described something incorrectly or have forgotten something important. We thank the participants for thinking about these ideas with us in such a wholehearted way. We hope that all of our therapy relationships are better for it. We also want to thank the Conference Collective for all the work they put into creating a conference where we can be in conversation with others about our commitments and those parts of our work closest to our hearts.

The first things that drew us to the work that is now called 'narrative therapy' were the therapeutic relationships that we witnessed in the work of Michael White and David Epston. Michael and David – as would be the case with any two people – related to people very differently from each other, and the relationships in each interview we saw were different. But something about the tone and feel of each of these relationships contrasted strongly with what we had previously thought of as 'therapeutic relationships'. They intrigued and excited us. They set us to dreaming about new things that might be possible for people who came to therapy, and about how our lives as therapists might be different if we could participate in such relationships.

Our years of working with narrative ideas and practices have only increased the appreciation we have for these ways of relating. Both the words and deeds of people we have worked with and our own experience show that 'narratively informed' therapy relationships offer possibilities for living that go beyond what we glimpsed in our early dreams.

It seems that certain ways of relating are presupposed in all narrative ideas, attitudes, and practices. However, they usually stay in the background – presumed, but not highlighted. As people who teach and write, we have long thought it might be useful to articulate ways of constituting narratively informed relationships. We don't mean to imply that our relationships are always exemplary. We thought, though, we might be able to participate with others in thinking about what goes into those therapy relationships we feel best about and what the people who come to consult with us find most helpful.

Writing with this in mind, we produced this first draft of a workshop description for the conference:

> *Exploration and conversation concerning how we might engage with other persons in open, caring, passionate, non-hierarchical, non-patronising 'therapy' relationships in which everyone can enact and embody their best aspirations, intentions, values, and visions, even though the dominant discourses of society attempt to frighten, restrain or oppress us every step of the way, or 'Is socially just love possible between therapists and the people who consult them?'*
>
> *We have witnessed some ways of relating that characterise the narrative work that moves us. Between now and February we will be*

thinking, planning, practising, and dreaming about how we might most usefully engage with others in an exploration of what might contribute to and constitute such relationships. We invite you to join us.

Even though we thought he might think the title was a little long and the body of the description a little short, we emailed this draft to David Denborough. Soon after we had clicked on the 'send' icon, our thoughts, plans, practice, and dreams began to be influenced by the voice of self-evaluation, which said, 'What do you mean non-hierarchical? There is always hierarchy. Wouldn't it be better to say 'minimise and/or expose hierarchy'?' 'Love? Do you really want to talk about love? People will think this is about being sappy or patronising. Are you implying that there is *a* narrative kind of relationship?'

We rewrote our description, using questions instead of statements. Then David's suggested revisions which, as always, helped us say what we intended to say even more clearly, arrived in our email box. With our description clarified, we began to shape the workshop itself. We decided that early on in our workshop we would let the work speak for itself by showing videotapes of two very different relationships that we believe show aspects of what a narratively informed therapeutic relationship might look like.

In one the work is very low key. I (GC) repeatedly ask the young person for his description of what is problematic. I am endeavouring to invite sincere collaboration, rather than capitulation or 'compliance'. The second shows a very emotional joining together in facing death. Many of the conventional 'rules' for therapeutic relationships are broken. It is a 'dual relationship' with someone who had previously come to study with us. I (JF) cry with the person I am working with. I also tell her about how I am changing through our relationship.

At the workshop, we asked participants as they watched our tapes to think about their own relationships so that we might all consider the following question throughout the three hours of the workshop: 'What are the effects of the relationships that we have on the work that we are joining together to do?'

After the two videotapes, we shared the list of questions that follows. We believe that these questions are useful in reflecting on, deconstructing, and revising the way we participate in relationships with the people who consult with us.

Questions we ask ourselves in cultivating narratively informed relationships

- Am I asking if and how the work is useful, and tailoring it in line with the response?
- Whose voice is being privileged in this relationship? What is the effect of that on the relationship and the work?
- Is anyone showing signs of being closed down, not able to fully enter into the work? If so, what power relations/ discourses are contributing to the closing down?
- What are we doing to foster collaboration? Among whom? What is the effect of that collaboration?
- Is this relationship opening up or closing down the experience of agency?
- Does this relationship take into account other relevant people, communities, and cultures? Are we considering the effects of the ripples of this relationship?

As we broke for lunch we asked these questions: 'What do these questions have you considering? What do you imagine asking yourself these questions would have you doing?'

After lunch we asked people to join us in a structure or exercise for thinking together about what narrative ideas and practices can bring to our relationships. Here we offer a version that is adapted so that it might work for a single reader. For those who appreciate thoroughness, we have broken it down into a lot of steps. If you like a brisker pace, you might try looking at only items 1, 2, 4, 6, 7, 9, & 11.

Structure for thinking about relationships

1. Think of a therapy relationship that you feel good about in relation to narrative ideas and values. You can pick a relationship that at times has exemplified a narratively informed relationship, even if at other times the relationship has not seemed narratively informed.

2. It may be useful to focus on a particular incident. These questions may help with that focus:
   When this relationship came to mind did you think of a particular incident?
   - Did you resolve a dilemma or hard place in a way that felt good to you?
   - At what point did you have the sense that the relationship was going in a direction that you felt good about?

3. At this point in the workshop, we asked people to turn to each other in pairs and take turns telling the story of whatever incident or event they had picked. You might find it makes the rest of this thought experiment richer to tell yourself the story of the incident you have picked – much as you would if you were telling it to someone else – before moving on.

4. Now, consider the incident or relationship you have chosen in terms of the attitudes, values, practices, and the like that are involved in it. You may find these questions helpful:
   - How did you pick this relationship or incident?
   - How would you describe it?
   - How would you characterise your position in relation to the people who came for help?
   - What practices were involved in bringing forth and maintaining the relationship?

5. At this time, you may want to write a list of some of the attitudes, values, practices, or intentions that seem to have been involved in the relationship.

6. Are you always fully pleased with the relationships you negotiate in your work? If you are willing, think for a moment now of a situation in which it was difficult to enter into the kind of relationship that you prefer. You might think about particular situations that brought on a sense of dread, of relationships that seemed restricted and thin, of people for whom you found yourself acting 'over-responsibly', or of a therapy relationship you just didn't feel good about. Identify such a situation, but please don't put yourself back in the middle of it.

7. Think about what got in the way. You might consider what could account for the sense of dread, restriction, over-responsibility or your less-than-good feelings about the relationship.

8. You might want to write down some of the ideas, discourses, institutions, or the like that got in the way.

9. Consider how one might undermine, oppose, ignore, or get around those difficulties and discourses. These questions might help:
   - If you had your 'self' from the preferred, narratively informed relationship and the other members of that relationship as a consulting team, what difference would it make when one or another of these difficulties or discourses threatens to take over a relationship?
   - Is there knowledge or experience from your preferred relationship that would be of help here?
   - If you were to take one small step in a preferred direction in regard to dealing with these difficulties or discourses, what would it be? What effects might it have if you take that step?

10. Take a few minutes to reflect on any thoughts, new ideas, or experiences that you had while considering the above questions.

11. Now consider one last question: 'Who stands beside you or could stand with you in being the person you want to be in this work and in having the kinds of relationships that you prefer?'

In Adelaide, once we had all gone through this exercise, we reflected on it as a large group. We heard some inspiring stories, and with the participants we developed the two lists that follow. While we have tried to include everything that was said, we have reduced some rich stories to a word or a short phrase – a pretty thin account. We apologise for the distortion that has inevitably crept in through this process. We invite you to add any items from your own list that you like. If you have listed things that are substantially different from what you see here, we'd love to hear from you.

Due to considerations of space and time, we will not discuss or explain any of what appears in the lists. Some of it will almost certainly be familiar to you. Some of it may not make sense. You may disagree with some items, or wonder what they have to do with narrative therapy. We hope that something on each list catches your interest or inspires you in some small way.

Some ideas, discourses, and practices that stand in the way of narratively informed relationships

- Certain constructions of 'Professionalism'
- Gender socialisation and discourses
- Certain constructions of expert knowledge
- Paternalism, including 'over-caring', 'over-concern', 'over-responsibility'
- Capitalism
- Upward accountability within hierarchies
- Time pressure
- Confusing people with their reputations
- The idea that therapeutic relationships are only about 'the client'
- Certain constructions of 'Boundaries'
- Certain constructions of 'Confidentiality'
- Classism
- Racism
- Ageism
- Degreeism
- Heterosexual dominance
- Therapy as the identification and correction of pathology
- Certain constructions of 'Neutrality'

Some practices and ideas that help subvert limiting discourses while supporting and encouraging narratively informed relationships

- Asking instead of assuming
- Naming and unpacking the practices and values involved in 'therapeutic relationships'
- Carrying teams with us in our hearts and minds
- Having conversations with colleagues about uncertainties and dilemmas
- Resisting compartmentalisation
- Asking questions we would like to be asked
- Externalising conversations
- Consulting those we work with as experts
- Collaborating
- Transparency/being public
- Situating, sharing relevant experiences
- Reflecting on and deconstructing the effects of our practices
- Decentring ourselves by using teams, leagues, and communities of concern
- Witnessing (outsider-witness groups and facilitating people hearing each other's stories during an interview)
- Inquiring into preferred directions in life
- Learning from those we work with
- 'Taking it back' practices
- Rejoicing in (not believing we have to squelch) feelings
- Believing in people's skills and agency

- Consulting about the process – asking: 'How is this going for you? Am I missing something important? Is this what you want to be talking about?'
- Having an open heart. Loving those we work with. Showing that we care and being kind
- Having patience
- Being respectful
- Questioning and being willing to break from 'the rules'
- Taking part in practices that involve people in more privileged/powerful positions being accountable to those in less privileged/powerful positions

We left this workshop with the sense that we had gained a very large team that we can join with in forging new ground for our relationships in the future. We invite you to join as well.

Note

1. This exercise was originally published in *Dulwich Centre Journal,* 2000 Nos.1&2.

References

Adams-Westcott, J., Dafforn, T. & Sterne, P. 1993: 'Escaping victim life stories and co-constructing personal agency.' In S. Gilligan & R. Price (eds), *Therapeutic Conversations* (pp.258-271). New York: Norton.

Andersen, T. 1987: 'The reflecting team: Dialogue and metadialogue in clinical work.' *Family Process*, 26:415-428.

Andersen, T. (ed) 1991: *The Reflecting Team: Dialogues and dialogues about the dialogues.* New York: Norton.

Anderson, H. & Goolishian, H. 1988: 'Human Systems as linguistic systems: Preliminary and evolving ideas about the implications for clinical theory.' *Family Process*, 27(4):371-393.

Anderson, H. & Goolishian, H. 1990: 'Beyond cybernetics: Comments on Atkinson and Heath's "Further thoughts on second-order family therapy".' *Family Process*, 29(2):157-163.

Anderson, H. & Goolishian, H. 1992: 'The client is the expert: A not-knowing approach to therapy.' In S. McNamee & K.J. Gergen (eds), *Therapy as Social Construction* (pp.25-39). Newbury Park, CA: Sage.

Anderson, W.T. 1990: *Reality Isn't What It Used To Be: Theatrical politics, ready-to-wear religion, global myths, primitive chic, and other wonders of the postmodern world.* San Francisco: Harper & Row.

Avis, J.M. 1985: 'The politics of functional family therapy: A feminist critique.' *Journal of Marital and Family Therapy,* 11:127-138.

Bailey, C.E. PhD (ed) 2000: *Children in Therapy: Using the family as a resource.* New York: Norton.

Bateson, G. 1972: *Steps to an Ecology of Mind.* New York: Ballantine Books.

Belenky, M.F., Clinchy, B.M., Goldberger, N.R. & Tarule, J.M. 1986: *Women's Ways of Knowing.* New York: Basic Books.

Berger, P. & Luckmann, T. 1966: *The Social Construction of Reality.* New York; Doubleday.

Boscolo, L. & Bertrando, P. 1992: 'The reflexive loop of past, present, and future in systemic therapy and consultation.' *Family Process,* 31(2):119-130.

Brooks, P. 1984: *Reading For Phi: Design and intention in narrative.* New York: Knopf.

Bruner, E. 1986: 'Ethnography as narrative.' In V. Turner & E. Bruner (eds), *The Anthropology of Experience.* Chicago: University of Illinois Press.

Bruner, E. 1986: 'Experience and its expressions.' In E. Bruner & V. Turner (eds), *The Anthropology of Experience* (pp.3-20). Chicago: University of Illinois Press.

Bruner, J. 1986: *Actual Minds/Possible Worlds.* Cambridge, MA: Harvard University Press.

Bruner, J. 1990: *Acts of Meaning.* Cambridge: Harvard University Press.

Bruner, J. 1991: 'The narrative construction of reality.' *Critical Inquiry,* 18:1-21.

Carter, E., Papp, P., Silverstein, O. & Walters, M. 1984: *Mothers and Sons, Fathers and Daughters* (monograph series, Vol.2 No.1). Washington, DC: The Women's Project in Family Therapy.

Cecchin, G. 1987: 'Hypothesizing, circularity, and neutrality revisited: An invitation to curiosity.' *Family Process,* 26:405-413.

Cohen, S.M., Combs, G., DeLaurenti, B., DeLaurenti, P., Freedman, J., Larimer, D. & Shulman, D. 1998: 'Minimizing hierarchy in therapeutic relationships: A reflecting team approach.' In M. Hoyt (ed), *Handbook of Constructive Therapies: Innovative approaches from leading practitioners* (pp.276-293). San Francisco: Jossey-Bass.

Combs, G.& Freedman, J. 1990: *Symbol, Story, and Ceremony: Using metaphor in individual and family therapy.* New York: Norton.

Combs, G. & Freedman, J. 1994: 'Narrative intentions.' In M.F. Hoyt (ed), *Constructive Therapies* (pp.67-91). New York: Guilford Press.

Combs, G. & Freedman, J. 1998: 'Tellings and retellings.' *Journal of Marital and Family Therapy,* 4:405-408.

Combs, G. & Freedman, J. 2000: 'Narrative therapy with couples.' In Dattilio, F.M. & Bevilacqua, L. (eds), *Comparative Treatments for Relationship Dysfunction.* New York: Springer.

Derrida, J. 1988: *Limited Inc.* Evanston, IL: Northwestern University Press.

Dickerson, V. 1996: 'On the client's voice.' *AFTA Newsletter,* 64:10.

Dickerson, V.C. & Zimmerman, J.L. 1993: 'A narrative approach to families with adolescents.' In S. Friedman (ed.), *The New Language of Change; Constructive collaboration in psychotherapy* (pp.226-250). New York: Guilford Press

Doan, R. & Clifton, D. 1990: 'The rules of problem lifestyles: Making externalizations more real.' *Dulwich Centre Newsletter,* 4:18.

Dugan, T. & Coles. R. 1989: *The Child In Our Times: Studies in the development of resiliency.* New York: Brunner/Mazel.

Durrant, M. 1989: 'Temper taming: An approach to children's temper problems revisited.' *Dulwich Centre Newsletter,* Autumn, pp.3-11.

Durrant, M. 1995: *Creative Strategies for School Problems.* New York: Norton.

Durrant, M. & Kowalski, K. 1990: 'Overcoming the effects of sexual abuse: Developing a self-perception of competence.' In M. Durrant & C. White (eds), *Ideas for Therapy with Sexual Abuse.* Adelaide, Australia: Dulwich Centre Publications.

De Shazer, S. 1991: *Putting Difference to Work.* New York: Norton.

Eisler, R. 1987: *The Chalice and the Blade: Our history, our future.* New York: Harper & Row.

Epston, D. 1989: *Collected Papers.* Adelaide, Australia: Dulwich Centre Publications.

Epston, D. 1992: 'Temper tantrum parties: Saving face, losing face, or going off your face.' In D. Epston & M. White, *Experience, Contradiction, Narrative, and Imagination: Selected papers of David Epston and Michael White, 1989-1991.* Adelaide, Australia: Dulwich Centre Publications.

Epston, D. 1993: 'Internalized other questioning with couples: The New Zealand version.' In S. Gilligan & R. Price (eds), *Therapeutic Conversations* (pp.183-189). New York: Norton.

Epston, D. 1993: 'Internalizing discourses versus externalizing discourses.' In S. Gilligan & R. Price (eds), *Therapeutic Conversations* (pp.161-177). New York: Norton.

Epston, D. 1998: *Catching up with David Epston: A collection of narrative practice-based papers published between 1991 and 1996.* Adelaide, Australia: Dulwich Centre Publications.

Epston, D. 1999: 'Co-research: The making of an alternative knowledge.' In *Narrative Therapy and Community Work: A conference collection* (pp.137-157). Adelaide, Australia: Dulwich Centre Publications.

Erickson, M.H. c.1930/1980: 'Shock and surprise facilitating a new self-image.' In E.L. Rossi (ed), *The Collected Papers of Milton H. Erickson on Hypnosis. IV. Innovative hypnotherapy* (pp.482-490). New York: Irvington.

Erickson, M.H. 1953: 'The therapy of a psychosomatic headache.' *Journal of Clinical and Experimental Hypnosis,* (4):2-6.

Erickson, M.H. 1965/1980: 'The use of symptoms as an integral part of hypnotherapy.' In E.L. Rossi (ed), *The Collected Papers of Milton H. Erickson on hypnosis. IV. Innovative hypnotherapy* (pp.212-223). New York: Irvington.

Erickson, M.H. & Rossi, E.L. 1979: *Hypnotherapy: An exploratory case book.* New York: Irvington.

Erickson, M.H. & Rossi, E.L. 1981: *Experiencing Hypnosis: Therapeutic approaches to altered states.* New York: Irvington.

Erickson, M.H., Rossi, E., & Rossi, S. 1976: *Hypnotic Realities: The induction of clinical hypnosis and forms of indirect suggestion.* New York: Irvington.

Foucault, M. 1965: *Madness and Civilization: A history of insanity in the age of reason.* (R. Howard, trans.) New York: Random House.

Foucault, M. 1975: *The Birth of the Clinic: An archeology of medical perception.* (A.M. Sheridan Smith, trans.) New York: Random House.

Foucault, M. 1977: *Discipline and Punish: The birth of the prison.* (A. Sheridan, trans.) New York: Pantheon Books.

Foucault, M. 1980: *Power/Knowledge: Selected interviews and other writings, 1972-1977.* (C. Gordon, ed.) New York: Pantheon Books.

Foucault, M. 1985: *The History of Sexuality, Vol. 2: The use of pleasure.* (R. Hurley, trans.) New York: Pantheon Books.

Freedman, J. 1999: 'Bringing it back to practice' *Dulwich Centre Journal* No.4.

Freedman, J. & Combs, G. 1993: 'Invitations to new stories: Using questions to explore alternative possibilities.' In S. Gilligan & R. Price (eds), *Therapeutic Conversations* (pp.291-303). New York: Norton.

Freedman, J. & Combs, G. 1994: 'Narrative intentions.' In M. Hoyt (ed), *Constructive Therapies,* (pp.291-303). New York: Guilford Press.

Freedman, J. & Combs, G. 1996a: *Narrative Therapy: The social construction of preferred realities.* New York: Norton.

Freedman, J. & Combs, G. 1996b: 'Gender stories.' *Journal of Systemic Therapies,* 75(1):31-46.

Freedman, J. & Combs, G. 1997: 'Lists.' In C. Smith & D. Nylund (eds), *Narrative Therapies with Children and Adolescents* (pp.147-161). New York: Guilford Press.

Freedman, J. & Combs, G. 2000: 'Therapy relationships that open possibilities for us all.' *Dulwich Centre Journal,* 1&2:17-20.

Freeman, J., Epston, D. & Lobovits, D. 1997: *Playful Approaches to Serious Problems: Narrative therapy with children and families.* New York: Norton.

Friedman, S. (ed) 1995: *The Reflecting Team in Action: Collaborative practice in family therapy.* New York: Guilford Press.

Garbarino, J., Dubrow, N., Kostelny, K. & Pardo, C. 1992: *Children in danger: Coping with the consequences of community violence.* San Francisco: Jossey-Bass.

Geertz, C. 1978: *The Interpretation of Cultures.* New York: Basic Books.

Geertz, C. 1983: *Local Knowledge.* New York: Basic Books.

Geertz, C. 1986: 'Making experiences, authoring selves.' In V. Turner & E. Bruner (eds), *The Anthropology of Experience.* Champaign: University of Illinois Press.

Gergen, K.J. 1985: 'The social constructionist movement in modern psychology.' *American Psychologist,* 40(3):266-275.

Gergen, K.J. 1991: *The Saturated Self: Dilemmas of identity in contemporary life.* New York; Basic Books.

Gilligan, C. 1982: *In a Different Voice: Psychological theory and women's development.* Cambridge, MA: Harvard University Press.

Gilligan, C. 1993: Statement made in presentation at the *Learning From Women Conference*, April. Boston, MA.

Goldner, V. 1985a: 'Feminism and family therapy.' *Family Process,* 24:31-47.

Goldner, V. 1985b: 'Warning: Family therapy may be dangerous to your health.' *The Family Therapy Networker,* 9:19-23.

Goodrich, T.J. 1991: 'Women, power, and family therapy: What's wrong with this picture?' *Journal of Feminist Therapy,* 3:5-37.

Griffith, J. & Griffith, M. 1994: *The Body Speaks.* New York: HarperCollins.

Gurman, A.S. & Jacobson, N.S. (eds) 2002: *Clinical Handbook of Couple Therapy* (3rd edition). New York. Guilford Press.

Haley, J. 1973: *Uncommon Therapy: The psychiatric techniques of Milton H. Erickson, M.D.* New York: Norton.

Hall, R. 1996: 'Partnership Accountability' in McLean, C., Carey, M., & White, C. (eds), *Men's Ways of Being*. Boulder, Colorado: Westview Press.

Hare-Mustin, R. 1978: 'A feminist approach to family therapy.' *Family Process,* 17:181-194.

Hare-Muslin, R. 1987: 'The problem of gender in family therapy theory.' *Family Process,* 26:15-27.

Hare-Mustin, R. 1991: 'Sex, lies, and headaches: The problem is power.' *Journal of Feminist Family Therapy,* 3:39-61.

Hare-Mustin, R. 1994: 'Discourses in the mirrored room: A postmodern analysis of therapy.' *Family Process,* 33(1):19-35.

Hoffman, L. 1990: 'Constructing realities: An art of lenses.' *Family Process,* 29:1-12. Laird, J. 1989: 'Women and stories: Restorying women's self-constructions.' In M. McGoldrick, C. Anderson, & F. Walsh (eds), *Women in Families: A framework for family therapy* (pp.427-450). New York: Norton.

Hoffman, L. 1991: 'Foreword.' In T. Andersen (ed), *The Reflecting Team: Dialogues and dialogues about the dialogues* (pp.ix-xiv). New York: Norton.

Hoyt, M.F. & Combs, G. 1996: 'On ethics and the spiritualities of the surface: A conversation with Michael White.' In M.F. Hoyt (ed), *Constructive Therapies* (Vol.2, pp.33-59). New York: Guilford Press.

Jackson, S. 2002: 'Self-forgiveness' *The International Journal of Narrative Therapy and Community Work,* No.1.

Kamsler, A. 1990: 'Her-story in the making: Therapy with women who were sexually abused in childhood.' In M. Durrant & C. White (eds), *Ideas for Therapy with Sexual Abuse.* Adelaide, Australia: Dulwich Centre Publications.

LaFollette, H. 1992: 'Real men.' In L. May & R. Strikwerda (eds), *Rethinking Masculinity: Philosophical explorations in light of feminism* (pp.59-74). Lanham, MD: Littlefield Adams Quality Paperbacks.

Laird, J. 1989: 'Women and stories: Restorying women's self-constructions.' In M. McGoldrick, C. Anderson & F. Walsh (eds), *Women in Families: A framework for family therapy* (pp.427-450). New York: Norton.

Leonard, L. 1982: *The Wounded Woman: Healing the father-daughter relationship.* Athens, OH: Swallow Press.

Loptson, C. & Stacey, K. 1995: 'Children should be seen and not heard? Questioning the unquestioned.' *Journal of Systemic Therapies,* 14(4):16-32.

Lowe, R. 1991: 'Postmodern themes and therapeutic practices: Notes towards the definition of Family Therapy: Part 2.' *Dulwich Centre Newsletter* (3):41-52.

MacCormack, T. & Tomm, K. 1998: 'Social constructionist/narrative couple therapy.' In F.M. Dattilio (ed), *Case Studies in Couple and Family Therapy: Systemic and cognitive perspectives* (pp.303-330). New York: Guilford Press.

Madigan, S.P. 1993: 'Questions about questions: Situating the therapist's curiosity in front of the family.' In S.G. Gilligan & R. Price (eds), *Therapeutic Conversations* (pp.219-230). New York: Norton.

Madigan, S. 1996: 'Undermining the problem in the privatization of problems in persons: Considering the socio-political and cultural context in the externalizing of internalized problem conversations.' *Journal of Systemic Therapies,* 5:47-62.

Maisel, R. 1994: *Engaging Men in a Re-evaluation of Practices and Definitions of Masculinity.* Paper presented at the Narrative Ideas and Therapeutic Practice Conference, April. Vancouver, British Colombia.

McLean, C. 1992: 'Introduction.' Some thoughts on men's ways of being. *Dulwich Centre Newsletter,* 3&4:3-8.

McLean, C. 1995: 'Boys and education in Australia.' *Dulwich Centre Newsletter,* 1&2:29-42.

McLean, C., Carey, M., & White, C. 1996: 'Introduction.' In McLean, C., Carey, M., & White, C. (eds), *Men's Ways of Being*. Boulder, Colorado: Westview Press.

Mead, M. 1977: 'The originality of Milton Erickson.' *American Journal of Clinical Hypnosis,* 20(l):4-5.

Monk, G., Winslade, J., Crocket, K. & Epston, D. (eds) 1997: *Narrative Therapy in Practice: The archeology of hope.* San Francisco: Jossey-Bass.

Morgan, A. 1995: 'Taking responsibility: Working with teasing and bullying in schools.' *Dulwich Centre Newsletter,* 2&3:16-28.

Morgan, A. 2000: *What is Narrative Therapy? An easy-to-read introduction.* Adelaide, Australia: Dulwich Centre Publications.

Myerhoff, B. 1982: 'Life history among the elderly: Performance, visibility, and remembering.' In J. Ruby (ed), *A Crack in the Mirror: Reflexive perspectives in anthropology* (pp.99-117). Philadelphia: University of Pennsylvania Press.

Myerhoff, B. 1986: 'Life not death in Venice: Its second life.' In V. Turner & E. Bruner (eds), *The Anthropology of Experience* (pp.261-285). Chicago: University of Illinois Press.

Radke-Yarrow, M., Zahn-Waxler, C. & Chapman, M. 1983: 'Children's prosocial dispositions and behavior.' In P.H. Mussen (ed), *Handbook of Child Psychology, Vol. IV: Socialization, personality, and social development* (4th ed.). New York; Wiley.

Reiss, D. 1985: 'Commentary: The social construction of reality - the passion within us all.' *Family Process,* 24:254-257.

Rorty, R. 1989: *Contingency, Irony, and Solidarity.* New York: Cambridge University Press.

Rorty, R. 1991: *Essays on Heidegger and Others: Philosophical papers, Vol.2.* New York: Cambridge University Press.

Rosen, S. 1982: *My Voice Will Go With You: The teaching tales of Milton H. Erickson.* New York: Norton.

Roth, S. & Epston, D. 1996a: 'Consulting the problem about the problematic relationship: An exercise for experiencing a relationship with an externalized problem.' In M. Hoyt (ed), *Constructive Therapies* (Vol.2, pp.148-162). New York: Guilford Press.

Roth, S. & Epston, D. 1996b: 'Developing externalizing conversations: An exercise.' *Journal of Systemic Therapies,* 15(l):5-12.

Ryle, G. 1990/1971: *Collected Papers: Critical essays and collected essays 1929-68.* Bristol, UK: Thoemmes Press. (Original work published 1971.)

Seligman, M., Revick, K., Jaycox, L. & Gillham, J. 1995: *The Optimistic Child.* New York: Harper & Row.

Stacey, K. 1995: 'Language as an exclusive or inclusive concept: Reaching beyond the verbal.' *Australian & New Zealand Journal of Family Therapy,* 76(3):123-132.

Taggart, M. 1985: 'The feminist critique in epistemological perspective: Questions of context in family therapy.' *Journal of Marital and Family Therapy,* 11:113-126.

Tamasese, K. & Waldegrave, C.1994: 'Cultural and gender accountability in the 'just therapy' approach' *Dulwich Centre Newsletter,* Nos 2&3.

Tamasese, K., Waldegrave, C. Tuhaka, F. & Campbell, W. 1998: 'Furthering conversation about partnerships of accountability: Talking about issues of leadership, ethics and care. *Dulwich Centre Journal.* No. 4

Tomm, K. 1988: 'Interventive interviewing: Part III. Intending to ask lineal, circular, strategic, or reflexive questions?' *Family Process,* 27(1):1-15.

Tomm, K. 1989: 'Externalizing the problem and internalizing personal agency.' *Journal of Strategic and Systemic Therapies,* 8(1):54-59.

White, M. 1984: 'Pseudo-encopresis: From avalanche to victory, from vicious to virtuous cycles.' *Family Systems Medicine,* 2(2):150-160.

White, M. 1986: 'Negative explanation, restraint and double description: A template for family therapy.' *Family Process,* 25:169-184.

White, M. 1987: 'Family therapy and schizophrenia: Addressing the "in-the-corner" lifestyle.' *Dulwich Centre Newsletter,* Spring, pp.14-21.

White, M. 1988: 'The process of questioning: A therapy of literary merit?' *Dulwich Centre Newsletter,* Winter, pp.8-14.

White, M. 1988/9: 'The externalizing of the problem and the re-authoring of lives and relationships.' *Dulwich Centre Newsletter,* Summer, pp.3-20.

White, M. 1989: 'Fear busting and monster taming: An approach to the fears of young children.' In M. White, *Selected papers.* Adelaide, Australia: Dulwich Centre Publications.

White, M. 1989: *Selected Papers.* Adelaide, Australia: Dulwich Centre Publications.

White, M. 1991: 'Deconstruction and therapy.' *Dulwich Centre Newsletter,* 3:21-40. Reprinted in S. G. Gilligan & R. Price (eds) 1993: *Therapeutic conversations* (pp.22-61). New York: Norton.

White, M. 1995: 'Reflecting teamwork as definitional ceremony.' In M. White, *Re-Authoring Lives: Interviews and essays* (pp.172-198). Adelaide, Australia: Dulwich Centre Publications.

White, M. 1995a: *Re-authoring lives: Interviews and essays.* Adelaide, Australia: Dulwich Centre Publications.

White, M. 1997: *Narratives of Therapists' Lives.* Adelaide, Australia: Dulwich Centre Publications.

White, M. 2000: *Reflections on Narrative Practice: Essays and interviews.* Adelaide, Australia: Dulwich Centre Publications.

White, M. & Epston, D. 1990: *Narrative Means to Therapeutic Ends.* New York: Norton.

White, M. & Epston, D. 1992: *Experience, Contradiction, Narrative, and Imagination.* Adelaide, Australia: Dulwich Centre Publications.

Zeig, J. 1980: *A Teaching Seminar with Milton H. Erickson.* New York: Brunner/Mazel.

Zeig, J. 1985: *Experiencing Erickson: An introduction to the man and his work.* New York: Brunner/Mazel.

Zeig, J. 1994: *Ericksonian Methods: The essence of the story.* New York: Brunner/Mazel.

Zimmerman, J.L. & Dickerson, V.C. 1994: 'Using a narrative metaphor: Implications for theory and clinical practice.' *Family Process,* 33:233-246.

Zimmerman, J. & Dickerson, V. 1996: *If Problems Talked: Narrative therapy in action.* New York: Guilford Press.